The Caregiver Resource Guide

Blessed are the Caregivers

Charles Puchta, CSA

2005 Edition

TABLE OF CONTENTS

1.	Getting Started	11
2.	Clarity in Purpose	37
3.	Lifestyle Planning	57
4.	Transportation Concerns	79
5.	Living Environments	91
6.	Care Options	113
7.	Legal Planning	129
8.	Government Programs	151
9.	Estate Matters	173
10.	End-Of-Life Planning	195
11.	The Talk	211
12.	Emotional Challenges	223
13.	Legacy of Memories	233
14.	Facing Death	243
15.	Closing Comments	257
16.	Key Terms and Definitions	259

#1

Getting Started

Everyone has dreams for his or her life and retirement years. The dreams are never to become dependent on someone else for the daily essentials of basic life. Caring for a loved one can be an extremely rewarding experience; however, at times it can be overwhelming, exhausting and depressing. There are no short cuts or easy answers, and every day is a new adventure. Family members may be eager to provide care and support for a parent or spouse, however, reaching agreements about the giving and receiving of care can be challenging. Likewise, it can be difficult to balance family, work and personal obligations.

Quite often it is a crisis situation that occurs and brings to your attention the need to provide care and support. Be careful. Making decisions in crisis can be challenging. Emotions can confuse the issues and options are seldom given the consideration they merit. The focus tends to be on the "here and now," trying to resolve the crisis, rather than focusing on solutions that make sense in the longer term.

Throughout this Resource Guide I provide practical knowledge that every family needs to know as loved ones age, become ill or face injury. While I use the terms "*Aging Parents*" and "*Loved Ones*" throughout the Resource Guide, the information is applicable whether a care receiver is a parent, spouse, friend or relative. Also, when referring to a care recipient, whether singular or plural, I generically use the pronouns "*he*" and "*she*." Please know that my intent is to be gender-neutral and the information applies whether the care recipient is male or female.

The Caregiver Resource Guide is released annually to ensure the information, perspectives and advice is current and up-to-date. The long-term care industry constantly changes based on research findings, emerging products and services, and changes in Government Programs, such as the Medicare Modernization Act of 2003. Let me get started by sharing three thought-provoking statements:

#1: *"People Simply Do The Best They Don't Know How"*

That's right; people do the best they <u>don't</u> know how. Make sure you understand this point. You don't do the best you know how, because if you have never dealt with issues involving aging and caregiving you probably have no idea what to expect and how to best help. So for those of you reading this book, congratulations! Seeking information and direction to help you along your journey is a critical step in the caregiving process. *The Caregiver Resource Guide* provides practical knowledge and unbiased information. I find that when families are aware of the issues, understand the options and alternatives, and recognize the implications of their actions and decisions, they are better able to make informed decisions. This leads to fewer regrets and being able to sleep better at night.

#2: *"People Don't Want To Care For an Aging Parent or Ill Spouse"*

When I say that we do not want to care for an aging parent or ill spouse, many people immediately take offense to this statement saying that in fact they do <u>want</u> to provide care. I'm not suggesting we are not <u>glad</u> to provide needed care. Instead I'm suggesting we would probably all prefer that our loved one not be in a position where care is necessary. In other words, we would prefer our loved ones to be living active and independent lifestyles where there has been no deviation from the wellness they might have enjoyed in their earlier years. Also, we would ideally like our loved ones to have sufficiently planned to meet any unexpected financial obligations due to aging or illness concerns. So the point is, if you had your choice of providing care or participating in a favorite hobby or pastime, we would probably all pick the latter.

#3: *"People Spend More Time 'Planning' When They Should be 'Preparing'"*

Again, I am drawing a distinction between two words to make a point. I find that most people spend time planning with they should be spending the time preparing. Why the distinction? Because invariably, plans seldom play out the way we expect. Planning is virtually impossible as there are too many variables outside of our control. For example, let's say at the age of 42, I develop my plan to retire at the age of 65 and to have saved $1,000,000. Well, what happens if I become ill at some point over the next 23 years? That wasn't part of my plan. What happens if the return on my investments are only 7.5% whereas my plan assumed a consistent 8.0%

return? That wasn't part of my plan. What if 23 years from now the Social Security award payments or Medicare benefits I receive are less than I expected? That wasn't part of my plan. You get the idea. My point is that while plans provide needed direction, they simply don't work. Instead, we need to prepare so that we are better able to make choices and informed decisions based on whatever situation we find ourselves in. The distinction I make is that people who plan, may only give consideration to, and plan for, the desired one option. People who prepare consider multiple options and are better able to respond in a variety of circumstances.

There Is No Escaping Caregiving

According to an editorial in the October 28, 2002 edition of The Cincinnati Enquirer entitled <u>Caregivers | Undervalued Resources,</u> *"Experts say 80 percent of us will be called on sometime in our lives to provide long-term care to parents, other relatives and friends. The value of these informal caregivers cannot be over estimated…They need medical, social and personal help because of chronic illnesses or disabilities, most often related to aging."*

The Kaiser Family Foundation estimates that there are more than 45 million family caregivers providing care to loved ones. According to an article in the Wall Street Journal entitled <u>For Some Parents, the Care Can't End</u> (7/2/02) an estimated 2.7 million adult children with developmental disabilities live at home with a family caregiver. One in four lives with a caregiver who is age 60 or older. The 2.7 million number reflects only developmental disabilities and does not include adult children with cancer, AIDS, Down syndrome, Huntington's, etc.

Former First Lady Rosalynn Carter sums it up best when she says: *"There are only four kinds of people in the world:*

- *Those who have been caregivers*
- *Those who currently are caregivers*
- *Those who will be caregivers*
- *Those who will need caregivers"*

(Source: The Rosalynn Carter Institute - http://rci.gsw.edu)

According to an article referencing a 2003 GE Center for Financial Learning Survey, published in the March 2004 SeniorResource.com ezine, *"45% of Americans have had a personal experience caring for an aging or ill*

13

relative." The article indicated that over 45% of the respondents who have had a personal caregiving experience have not taken steps to develop long-term care plans for themselves.

The lack of preparedness for caregiving is alarming. What I find astonishing is that while everyone is likely to be impacted by caregiving in one way or another, most people tend to spend more time planning for a vacation, than they do preparing for long-term care. Even people who have experienced caregiving first hand, and recognize the challenges and demands, resist personal planning.

Although everyone's situation is different, the basic challenges and predominant issues are usually the same. I find that people are better able to cope, and are more apt to act when they understand the issues with which they are dealing. Research that I have conducted over a five year period suggests that there are five main reasons caregivers find themselves overwhelmed and unprepared.

Top Five Reasons Why Caregiving is Challenging:

1. **INconsistent:** The age factor varies drastically as to when a person may face limitations or require assistance. Some people age gracefully and live independently into their 80's and 90's. Others face complications or illness in their 40's or 50's. This age inconsistency makes it difficult for families to know when to get more involved in a loved ones life, and when to begin considering aging and long-term care issues and options. Compounding this challenge is the fact that many people have a difficult time distinguishing between characteristics of normal aging from age related disease or illness. As a result, a person's condition often goes undiagnosed for a period of time before he or she receives the care and support needed and deserved.

2. **INdependent:** Family caregivers and persons needing or requiring assistance often do not seek support, as the issues they face tend to be personal and private. Family caregivers also find it difficult to identify, and as a result associate with, others facing similar challenges. The way many people approach caregiving is contrary to how we cope in day-to-day life. All through life, people find themselves part of naturally forming peer groups in their personal and professional lives. Regardless, people facing aging and illness related issues tend to isolate themselves and try to manage everything on their own instead of reaching out for help and direction.

3. **INexperienced**: It does not matter what you have done as an adult and parent, nothing has prepared you to deal with long-term care. Even medical professionals, who deal with patients' medical conditions on a daily basis, encounter unexpected emotional challenges when the concerned party is their loved one. Until people approach the age of 65, most have never given much consideration to anticipating health challenges, the receiving of care, navigating the Social Security and Medicare system, or the various other issues they are likely to encounter, let alone the thought of death.

4. **INtrusive:** All through life, people are taught to embrace the principles of 'Honor, Obey and Respect,' parents and elders. But, a common response to a family member who expresses concern or a wish to provide support is "*I'm fine.*" When that occurs, family members find themselves unsure how to respond, how to help and what to do. Another challenge can be the parent/child role reversal; even if a child recognizes a parent is unable to make rational decisions for himself.

5. **INterlocking:** There is a natural tendency to ask people questions specific to their experience or profession. For example, when you ask a doctor a question, you are likely to get an answer from a medical perspective. The problem is that the person asking the question is often expecting a Big Picture answer, not a response specific to a certain profession or viewpoint. Although it may be human nature to focus strictly on the problem or issue at hand, I find that by doing so, people often get blindsided by seemingly unrelated issues. That is why Aging America Resources takes the 'Big Picture' or 'Puzzle Piece' approach to helping people understand how the many lifestyle, administrative, emotional, and memorial issues are all interrelated.

The Big Picture

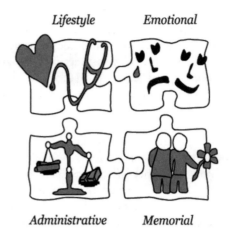

Lifestyle *Emotional*

Administrative *Memorial*

- **Lifestyle**: In this piece of the puzzle, I address day-to-day life issues such as a person's medical condition, functioning level (physical and mental), living environments, care needs, transportation, socialization, and nutrition.

- **Administrative**: This puzzle piece focuses on helping people coordinate their legal and financial affairs, and ensure family and friends are aware of and are prepared to address a loved one's wishes. I focus on advance directives, estate planning, Social Security, Medicare, Medicaid, life insurance, long-term care insurance, scams and having "The Talk."

- **Emotional**: The emotional piece of the puzzle covers the many heart and soul issues that people often overlook such as understanding the care recipient's perspective, coping, managing feelings, being confident in decision-making, and identifying and leveraging support resources.

- **Memorial**: In this piece of the puzzle I address not only end-of-life issues and considerations, but also things people can do to make the most of each day. I focus on preserving memories, generational planning, preparing for death, hospice care, what to do when a death occurs, funeral considerations and grieving.

Getting Started

The Big Picture Approach

My unique 'Big Picture' approach helps families understand, anticipate and address the predominant issues they may encounter as loved ones age or otherwise become incapacitated. I find that the natural tendency to focus on the 'issue at hand' often gives families a false sense of security. People often think that once they solve the immediate issue, they are done. They may not realize the next challenge could be moments or months away. As a result of not understanding how the four categories of issues are interrelated, people often get blindsided by unexpected issues. It can be helpful for families to look at aging and long-term care as a process, as opposed to an event.

Over the years, it has become apparent that care issues cannot be resolved in isolation. When a person focuses on an issue involving any of the four puzzle pieces, at least two other puzzle pieces are impacted.

For example, say your loved one is diagnosed with an illness (a Lifestyle issue). Because of a prognosis, many other Lifestyle issues may need to be addressed (e.g. Living Environment, Care Options, Transportation, etc.) But, before medical or care decisions can be made, families must understand the Administrative issues such as a loved one's wishes and expectations, who has legal authority, what type of insurance coverage is available, financial resources or limitations, and more. Families also encounter several Emotional issues that suddenly emerge, such as denial, sadness, guilt, or fear.

Likewise, at time of death, (a Memorial issue), there are associated Administrative issues such as estate matters, possibly surviving spouse concerns, and Emotional issues as you work through funeral arrangements, write an obituary, and memorialize your loved one's life.

As I reflect on the 10 years I spent caring for my parents, I think my biggest mistake was addressing each issue or task by itself. Although it felt right at the time, with each new challenge, we were not prepared. It was mentally and physically grueling! I wish my sister and I had known to consider the pieces of the puzzle and how everything is interrelated. While it may seem obvious now, it is not what people think about. For example, when my father was admitted into the hospital on his 79th birthday and the prognosis was not good, no one suggested we consider funeral planning until his death occurred.

Throughout the Resource Guide, I provide exercises that I encourage you to work through. Spreadsheets to support completing these exercises can be downloaded from the Internet in Microsoft Excel and Adobe PDF formats. Keep a hard copy of each worksheet accessible and in a safe place, so you can find it when you need it. To download an electronic copy of the worksheet templates, go to:

http://www.agingusa.com/2005worksheets.asp

Exercise #1: Personal Information

Start collecting basic information that you will inevitably need at a moments notice. For your sake, <u>do not</u> skip this exercise and come back to it later. The information you will want to capture includes the following:

EXERCISE #1 – Personal Information
Name (Legal):   Address: Telephone #'s (home, wireless):   Social Security #:   Medicare Claim #:
Place of Employment: (*If working*)   Address: Work Telephone #:   Supervisor's Name:
For each of the following medical professionals, indicate the specialty, Name, Address and Telephone #.   • Primary Care Physician: • Dentist: • Eye Doctor: • Podiatrist: • Specialist: (*e.g., Oncologist, Urologist, Gynecologist*):   • Specialist:
Primary Health Insurance Coverage: Provider: Policy #:   Contact Person (if any):   Telephone #:

Secondary or Supplemental Insurance: Type of Insurance: Insurance Company: Policy #: Contact Person (if any): Telephone #:
Other Insurance (e.g., Long Term Care): Type of Insurance: Insurance Company: Policy #: Agent's Name: Telephone #: Location of Original Policy:
Life Insurance: Type (*e.g. Term, Variable, etc.*): Insurance Company: Policy #: Agent's Name: Telephone #: Location of Original Policy:
Religious Affiliation: Place of Worship: Contact Name: Address: Telephone #:
Pharmacy: Address: Telephone #: Contact Person (if any):
Name of Financial Advisor: Name of Firm: Telephone #:
Name of Stock Broker: Name of Firm: Telephone #:
Primary Financial Institution: Branch Address:

Type of Account(s):
Account Number(s):
Contact Name:
Contact Telephone #:
Secondary Financial Institution:
Branch Address:
Type of Account(s):
Account Number(s):
Contact Name:
Contact Telephone #:
Location of Safety Deposit Box:
Safety Deposit Box Number:
Location of Safety Deposit Box Key:
Authorized Signatures:
Name of Attorney:
Name of Firm:
Telephone #:
Location of Advance Directives:
Person(s) Appointed Power of Attorney:
Driver's License #:
State of Issue:
Expiration Date:
Summary of Military Service:
Location Military Service Records:
Honors:
Location of Discharge Papers, etc.:
Location of Recent Tax Returns:
Credit Card Companies:
Account Holders Name (on each card):
Telephone #:
NOTE: Don't List Credit Card #'s.
Detail on in-force Service Contracts: (e.g. Alarm Monitoring, Pest Control, Lawn Service, etc.)
Detail on a pre-arranged or pre-paid Funeral Plans:
Location of written plans or contract:
Funeral Provider:
Contact Name:

Address:
Telephone #:
Location of Cemetery Plots:
Insurance Carriers for Auto, Home, Property & Casualty:
Company Name(s):
Telephone #'s:
Other:
Location of Vehicle Titles:
Location of Deed to House or other Real Estate:

This is not an exhaustive list. Add other information as your situation merits.

Common Starting Points

For most people reading this Resource Guide, one of three things has likely happened:

1. A life-changing event has occurred. (e.g. Illness, Hospitalization, Injury, Death of a Spouse)

2. Someone has come to realize or accept something that, up to this point, was not evident.

3. Someone is interested in planning ahead so they are prepared for the future.

To help you recognize the reality you may be facing, examples of each starting point are provided. With many people in denial regarding the situation and struggles a loved one may be facing, it can help to associate with one or more of the common starting points, and to realize you are not alone.

1. Life-changing Events:

- Diagnosis of a chronic debilitating disease (e.g., Alzheimer's, Parkinson's, Arthritis, Osteoporosis.)
- Diagnosis of terminal illness (e.g., Cancer.)
- Medical event (e.g. Heart Attack, Stroke.)
- Daily medication becomes required.
- Weekly doctor visit(s) becomes necessary.
- Oxygen or other support system becomes required.
- Walker, wheelchair or other assistive device becomes necessary.
- Hospitalization of one parent leaves the second parent home alone.

2. Realization on Your Part:

- Noticeable change in functional capabilities.
- Noticeable change in cognitive state.
- Noticeable change in activity level.
- Realization that daily tasks are becoming more difficult and time consuming (e.g., getting dressed, preparing a meal, balancing the checkbook.)
- Apprehension to try new things or venture outside familiar territory.

3. Planning Ahead: Often times people try to address a specific issue or topic such as:

- Knowing what signs to look for that may suggest functional challenges (physical and mental.)
- Understanding the various living environments and care options so that you are prepared if, or when, a change may be appropriate or necessary.
- Ensuring needed legal documents are executed and up-to-date.
- Understanding ones wishes, and the roles, responsibilities and expectations of family members.
- Developing a financial or retirement plan.
- Evaluating insurance coverage options.
- Creating a legacy of memories while still possible.

Regardless of which category most represents your situation, this Resource Guide will help you understand and address the issues you are likely to face and give you assurance to act with confidence.

Putting Aging Into Perspective

Aging is a fact of life. Whether facing the reality of turning 40, 50 or 60 years old or stepping into retirement, we all face the uncertainty of tomorrow. What is different about aging is that it tends to creep up on most people, and families do not know what to expect until they are there. Caregiving is also unique in that people's lives are impacted by the things families do, or do not do. Although there are many ways to provide care and assistance, caregivers often do not have the luxury of learning from their mistakes and "doing it better" or "trying harder" the next time.

Getting Started

On average, people are living longer. Longevity is expected to increase with advances in medical technology. Currently over 20% of America's population is over the age of 55. An estimated 35 million people are age 65 and older – one out of every eight people (12.5%) in America, and to many peoples surprise, the fastest growing segment of our population is people age 85 years and older. As our Baby Boomers age, the number of older adults (age 65+) is expected to double to 70 million over the next 20 years.

The average life expectancy for Americans is now at an all time high. The National Center for Health Statistics reports that the average life expectancy was 77.2 years in 2001, up by nearly two years since 1990. For women, the average life span was 79.8 years in 2001 and 74.4 years for men. In terms of ethnicity, the 1990 census data indicated that Caucasians lived an average of seven years longer than African-Americans.

The October 11, 2004 edition of Business Week magazine featured a story entitled *"Aging Is Becoming So Yesterday."* The story elaborated on how our bodies respond to the aging process and what we can expect. One caption from the story written by Catherine Arnst stated, *"The organs of the body suffer myriad indignities as we age, deteriorating in response to genetic signals and the wear and tear of daily life."* While the story offered insights into aging and the possibility of reengineering the body, what I found to be fascinating were the side-by-side photographs of Kirk Douglas. One picture showed him at age 30, next to that age 50, then age 72 and finally at age 88. As the saying goes, *"a picture is worth a thousand words."* Seeing the photographs brings reality to the aging process and makes denial more difficult.

While external and internal changes occur as people age, the external changes are most visible. External changes are the physical changes such as hair and skin. As early as our 30's and 40's, we notice changes to our hair color and the thickness of our hair, our skin begins to change, and wrinkles begin to appear. Other noticeable changes may have to do with eyesight, hearing, physical strength, balance and coordination. Internal changes are also happening. Our bodies become frailer, our minds may not be as sharp, we process and do things slower, we are more susceptible to illness, and our memory may fail. So, it is only reasonable that as loved ones age or become ill, family members should consider competency issues such as the following:

- Ability to live independently
- Ability to demonstrate sound judgment

- Ability to identify potentially dangerous situations
- Ability to manage finances
- Ability to administer medication

The following are some excerpts from an e-mail a friend recently sent me that helps put many day-to-day encounters into reality.

Have you ever noticed that when you are of a certain age, everything seems uphill from where you are? Stairs are steeper. Groceries are heavier. And, everything is farther away. Why is it, music is turned up louder and people are speaking more softly? Is there a conspiracy to try and make all the Baby Boomers a bunch of lip readers? Is it just me, or do people seem much younger than I was at the same age? And why is it that the people my own age appear so much older than I am?

The Advertising Effect

Many people are in denial about the realities of aging, and never give aging a thought until they find themselves facing a life changing event. When I look at brochures for organizations offering products to mature adults, it is no wonder. The photographs that appear always seem to show a beautiful silver haired couple walking on the beach at sunset, holding hands like there is not a worry in the world. Besides the images that make retirement look glamorous, people seem to deny aging in many other ways. Our society is so wrapped up in cosmetic surgery miracles, hair alterations and sexual performance enhancers that much of our culture no longer acknowledges aging, or even understands how to identify the aging process when it is happening right under our noses.

Aging is inevitable. In terms of the supposed Anti-Aging Industry and the many "Miracle Treatments", save your money. Scientist S. Jay Olshansky of the University of Illinois at Chicago says that *"anyone claiming that their product will slow, stop or reverse aging is lying."* Although many aspects of our health are beyond our control, we can reduce our chances of many problems by eating right, exercising regularly, maintaining a healthy weight, managing stress and having regular check-ups and health screenings. Also, beyond one's physical health, experts encourage people to regularly challenge their brains by reading, doing crossword puzzles or engaging in other mentally and intellectually stimulating exercises.

Getting Started

Successful Aging

According to the July 2002 Journal of the American Geriatrics Society (JAGS), maintaining one's physical functioning capacity and showing high cognitive abilities are essential elements of "Successful" or "Normal" Aging. Four predictors of successful aging are regular physical activity, social engagement, freedom from chronic illness and feeling of self-worth.

An article in the July 31, 2002 edition of The Cincinnati Enquirer entitled <u>Worried about getting older? Forget about it and be happy</u>, shares an interesting finding. The article focused on a report released from Researchers at Miami University (Ohio) and Yale University. *"A 23-year study found that those who had positive perceptions of aging lived an average of 7.5 years longer than those with cloudier outlooks."* So maybe attitude is more important than many people recognize.

Six Dimensions of Wellness

Regardless of one's age, the best medicine may be recognizing and addressing the following Six Dimensions of Wellness created by Dr. Bill Hettler. The way Dr. Hettler came to establish the Six Dimensions of Wellness is a fascinating human interest story. He was first introduced to the topic of wellness and health promotion in May of 1969 during the commencement exercise at his graduation from The University of Cincinnati College of Medicine.

The person offering the commencement address was a professor of Preventive Medicine, someone that most of the students had not seen before as his specialty had very little presence in the medical school curriculum. The speaker began by saying that "*You will save more lives, and alleviate more suffering if you never enter the practice of medicine.*" He went on to say that if they would spend their time <u>helping people learn how to live</u> instead of practicing traditional medicine, they would indeed save more lives and alleviate more suffering.

Over the years practicing medicine, Dr. Hettler realized that what people do for themselves in the way of lifestyle choices has a much greater impact on their chances of survival than anything physicians are likely to accomplish. For additional information on Dr. Hettler, visit his website at www.Hettler.com/sixdimen.htm. The six dimensions are as follows:

1. EMOTIONAL Wellness - refers to a person's emotions or feelings, and one's ability to manage stress and have satisfying relationships with others.

2. INTELLECTUAL Wellness - encourages stimulating one's mind or mental capacity to maintain and expand one's knowledge and skills.

3. OCCUPATIONAL Wellness - involves achieving personal satisfaction and enrichment from one's vocation.

4. PHYSCIAL Wellness - encourages activities to develop and maintain one's physical health with regular medical check-ups, self-care, physical exercise, proper nutrition, and the avoidance of drugs and excessive alcohol.

5. SOCIAL (Interpersonal) Wellness - fosters a positive self-image and encourages positive interactions in family and community.

6. SPIRITUAL Wellness - involves seeking and recognizing meaning and purpose in one's life and a spiritually centered belief system.

Aging and Caregiving Facts

As people live longer, there also comes a need to care for those who can not manage alone. An article from the February 10, 2004 edition of The Cincinnati Enquirer entitled <u>Old, infirmed turn to children,</u> by Francis X. Donnelly and Karen Bouffard (The Detroit News) referenced an interesting study. According to the AARP, "*the number of American households where residents care for aging relatives has more than tripled during the past decade, from 7 million to 22.4 million. The growing number reverberates through marriages, savings accounts and workplaces as people try to manage their parent's lives without losing control of their own.*" The article also said that while medical breakthroughs allow people to live longer, the quality of life is not always better.

As people reach the age of 65, there are several realities to consider. Studies say that 80% of the people age 65 or older are living with at least one (1) chronic illness. That illness could be Alzheimer's, arthritis, cancer, diabetes, osteoporosis, ALS, or some other medical condition. Studies also say that at least 35% of mature adults, those ages 65 and older, have three or more chronic health conditions. (Source: <u>Complete Guide to Aging and Health</u> – Williams, M.E.)

Someone with a chronic medical condition will face limitations. Family members and professionals serving mature clients need to be more aware and concerned. Whether challenges are mental, physical or psychological, many older adults will need assistance with their day-to-day affairs. The alternative is that people do not get the assistance they need and struggle unnecessarily.

It is important to clarify that 'getting' or 'accepting' help does not mean someone losses their independence or becomes dependent. With the advancements in the long-term care industry over the past 10 years, there are many options, programs and innovations that enable people to maintain their independence. Although nursing homes have long been thought to be the living environment of choice for today's seniors, the fact is that far fewer live in nursing homes than most people expect. It is estimated that just over 1% of people age 65–74 live in a nursing home at any given time. For folks age 75-84, the number is just shy of 5%. And, of those people age 85 and older, greater than 80% either live with family or alone (Source: US Senate Special Committee on Aging)

As our population ages and people become less independent, it is often a family member that steps in to help. What begins as a kind gesture or a helping hand often leads to more routine and extensive care. People expect to be needed part-time, but for many, the need eventually becomes full-time.

One of my favorite advertisements is for SunRise Assisted Living facilities. (http://www.SunRiseAssistedLiving.com) (*I am not endorsing this community; rather, I am giving them credit for their fabulous ad.*) The ad featured a picture of an elderly lady's face and the headline read *"Every line tells a story"* referring to the lines on her face. The wording went on to say *"Every hard earned line is a legacy and a lesson to us all."* What a great perspective and outlook. Be sure to respect, look out for, and up to, our elders.

What Is A Caregiver?

According to the Family Caregiver Alliance (www.caregiver.org) *"A caregiver is anyone who provides assistance to someone else that is in some degree incapacitated and needs help."* Someone who provides assistance is considered either a "formal" or "informal" caregiver. The term "formal" caregiver refers to a paid caregiver providing non-medical or medical care and may be professionally trained and certified. The term "informal" caregiver refers to an unpaid family member, friend or neighbor who provides either full-time or part-time care.

Other organizations suggest that a person crosses over into the caregiver role once they consistently spend a certain number of hours a week in a capacity where they are providing some sort of care or support. Whether the number is 2 hours or 12 hours, the point remains the same. It is important for people to recognize themselves as caregivers. I find that until an individual considers herself a caregiver, she may be reluctant to reach out for information, advice and support.

Other Facts of Interest

- In the last 100 years, the average life span of Americans jumped from 49 to 77. (Source AARP)
- The average person lives 15 years longer than those just one generation ago. (Source: Chicago Caregiver Magazine – March 2003)
- Family caregivers provide about 80% of the care for people who need help with daily activities (Source: AARP)
- An estimated 45 million unpaid, untrained family members provide care to loved ones. (Source: Kaiser Family Foundation, 2002)
- An estimated one in four households (22.4 million) is providing care to a person(s) age 50 or older. (Source: 1997 study of the National Alliance for Caregiving and the AARP)
- An estimated 22% of persons aged 45 to 55 are caring for, or are financial supporting, older relatives. (Source: Ibid)
- The number of households providing care is expected to increase to 39 million by 2007. (Source: Ibid)
- Over half of all informal caregivers are employed full-time elsewhere. (Source: Ibid)
- Roughly 30% of working people are caring for aging relatives. That figure is projected to rise to 54% by 2009, according to the US Department of Labor.
- The average caregiver is a 46-year-old woman who is married and is employed outside the home. (Source: National Alliance for Caregiving)

- Caregivers of people age 50+ spend about 18 hours a week providing care. The hours spent providing care to people age 65+ increases to over 20 hours. (Source: Ibid)

- 20% of the people caring for a family member or friend aged 50+ spend over 40 hours a week providing care, with some providing constant care. (Source: Ibid)

- Informal caregivers tend to provide unpaid assistance for between one and four years with an estimated 20% providing care for 5 years or longer. (Source: Ibid)

- Nearly seven (7) million Americans are long distance caregivers meaning that they travel at least one hour to perform their caregiving responsibilities. (Source: National Council on Aging.)

The following Dear Abby column, entitled <u>Relatives in denial; mom needs support,</u> appeared in the January 20, 2004 of The Cincinnati Enquirer. This article indicates the common struggles and thinking people often face.

"For years now, my dad's health has slowly deteriorated. He has good days when he kind of knows what's going on, and bad days when his whole world is off balance. Recently, he suffered some mini strokes, and last September the doctor diagnosed him with Alzheimer's.

I was there when Dad was diagnosed. You could see the look of relief on his face to finally have a name for what was going on inside him. He told the doctor, "Well at least now I know I'm not going crazy."

The problem is his siblings. They get angry at Mom when she tells the doctor how Dad is at home and accuse her of exaggerating. They get upset with us for not letting Dad drive, even though he doesn't see well and has been known to get lost. They have even gone behind out backs and told Dad he doesn't have Alzheimer's, which only compounds the problem.

...Poor mom has a hard enough time being a caregiver to a man who doesn't always recognize us and can't remember names."

RESPONSE: *...Your father's siblings are in deep denial – which is probably why they can't bring themselves to admit what is really happening. Their anger at your mother is part of their denial. They would rather believe that she is exaggerating than come to grips with the truth...."*

The reality is that denial is rampant. According to a SNAPSHOT® in the April 16, 2002 edition of the USA Today entitled <u>Alzheimer's often confused with aging</u>, Dementia is not a normal part of aging. Although the article is specific to a study on Alzheimer's, I believe the findings are relevant regardless of the disease. *"On average, Alzheimer's patients don't receive medical attention until one year after experiencing symptoms."* Percentage of caregivers who blame delay on: Fear of Diagnosis (9%), Denial (31%), Confusion with normal signs of aging (57%). (Source: Harris Interactive for Novartis Pharmaceuticals Corp. and the National Family Caregiver Association.)

Is It Time To Get Involved?

Having highlighted some of the common challenges, encouraged you to collect personal information, and provided some perspectives and facts on aging and caregiving; I suggest several considerations to help you and your family determine your level of involvement.

Regardless if a person is elderly, recovering from an illness or injury, or otherwise needs assistance, the challenges are often the same. There are some considerations and competencies that you should assess to determine if it might be appropriate to take a more active role in a loved one's life. Most people that face health-related challenges or limitations will not ask for help, as they tend to place a high value on their privacy and independence. Most people also do not want to be a burden to their family and friends.

Have you heard the saying, *"You are too close to the forest to see the trees?"* That concept applies to caregiving as well. People that frequently visit with loved ones often have a more difficult time recognizing or coming to grips with any deterioration in a loved one's functioning. Think about it. If you do not see someone for a long period the changes are more obvious than when you see someone daily. Regardless of the frequency you see someone; most people do not know what things they should look for to determine if it might be time to get more involved in a loved one's life.

I developed the following list of 10 considerations to help families and friends quickly assess a loved one's condition, and identify potential areas of concern. I suggest that if have any concerns, even with one issue, it may be time to take a more active role in a loved one's life. Chances are that your loved one may be struggling unnecessarily and it might be time to explore ways to help in a 'proactive' fashion, rather than waiting to react. Depending on the severity of your concerns, you may also want to seek professional advice.

Review the 10 Caregiving Considerations below and determine if it might be time for you to get more involved and help a loved one address challenges they may be facing.

1. <u>MEDICAL CONDITION</u> – Has your loved one been diagnosed with a disease, illness or other medical condition that could impact their daily living? How is the medical condition likely to cause limitations to a person's abilities now or in the future?

2. <u>DRIVING</u> - If your loved one drives, is there reason to believe they pose an above average risk for being involved in an accident? How are their reflexes, vision and ability to respond in an unexpected situation? Are they likely to get lost and panic?

3. <u>FOOD/NUTRITION</u> – Is your loved one eating balanced meals? Is their weight stable? Are they able to prepare meals? Are they able to manage grocery shopping? Do they have a reasonable variety of food in the refrigerator (with future expiration dates)?

4. <u>HYGIENE</u> - How does your loved one look and smell - including their breath? Does it appear they are bathing regularly? How are their overall appearance, grooming and ability to match clothing compared to prior years? Do their bed linens and bath towels appear clean? Are they able to manage the laundry?

5. <u>BEHAVIOR</u> – Does your loved one seem anxious or irritable? Does being away from home make them uncomfortable? Do they seem depressed? Are they inconsistent in the things they say? Does your loved one remember names, places and current events?

6. <u>DAILY TASKS</u> - Are basic tasks overly challenging, frustrating or time consuming for your loved one?   (example: getting ready to go out, preparing a meal or shopping.)

7. <u>MEDICATION</u> - Can your loved one manage their medications properly including dosage, frequency and changes to prescriptions? Do they understand why they are taking the medications? Are prescriptions getting refilled in a timely fashion?

8. <u>FINANCES</u> – Does it appear that your loved one is capable of making sound financial decisions? Are they able to manage their personal finances? Are bills being paid in a timely fashion? Do they have a reasonable amount of cash on hand?

9. <u>MAIL</u> - Is the mail stacking up? Do you see any past due or delinquency notices? Does your loved one appear to be a target for solicitation offers?

10. <u>SAFETY</u> – Is your loved one careful about turning off appliances (example: stove, coffee pot)? Do they ever carelessly leave candles or cigarettes burning? Are sharp objects properly put away? Do they keep the doors and windows locked – and are they able to locate the keys?

Whenever possible, try to observe your loved one in a variety of situations. Ideally, this evaluation should be informal, so as not to cause alarm or appear disrespectful. If you have a concern, even with one area, chances are that your loved one may be struggling unnecessarily. Trust your instincts.

We suggest you and your family begin by acknowledging any areas of concern and start to learn about the issues and options available. Conversations should reflect a partnership and demonstrate a willingness to work together. Let your loved one know your intent is to understand and respect their wishes while providing for their needs. (See Chapter #11 entitled The Talk.)

Often there are simple things you can do to provide assistance. I encourage you not to wait until a medical diagnosis or a crisis situation occurs before you begin to consider to the issues and challenges a loved one may face. In the following chapters, I elaborate on things you might consider doing to address potential areas of concern. For example:

• MEDICAL CONDITION - Go with your parent or loved one to his next doctor's appointment and hear first hand what the doctor has to say. It is not uncommon for an older person to avoid asking questions as he might not want to hear what the doctor has to say, or he might not be able to process and understand what is being said.

• DRIVING - If your parent drives, let him drive when you go out to lunch or run an errand. Observe his driving skills and determine if his abilities present concerns. If you have concern, learn about the programs and alternatives that might be appropriate.

- FOOD / NUTRITION – Offer to help with grocery shopping, make an extra casserole each week for a loved one, or look into organizations and programs that might deliver meals.

- HYGIENE – If towels, linens or clothes do not appear fresh, offer to do an occasional load of laundry or suggest outside assistance. Often tasks that may be easy for a younger person may be more challenging to others. Do not assume. Ask how you can help.

- BEHAVIOR – If a person is showing unusual behavior, try to determine if there are certain times of the day or situations where the behaviors are more extreme. If there are situations that cause anxiety such as crowds and noise (e.g. over stimulation), try to avoid them. Provide reassurance to the person that *"It's going to be okay"* and seek medical help as you deem appropriate.

- DAILY TASKS – Determine if there might be daily tasks that you can perform to help lighten the load. Also, give consideration to the ability and comfort level of people to perform tasks. Especially in the case where one spouse suddenly finds herself alone, she may not be comfortable handling certain tasks.

- MEDICATIONS – See if there might be ways to help with medications such as sorting pills into day of the week dispensers. Also consider placing reminders in the house or making a reminder phone call. Keep a list of all medications, the purpose, prescribing medical professional, and expected refill date.

- FINANCES – Keeping up-to-date on finances can be difficult for some people. With advances like internet banking and automatic bill payment services, maybe a family member can provide assistance.

- MAIL – Typical behaviors with the US Mail seem to change as people age. What might have once been considered junk mail is often opened and kept. I suggest family members warn loved ones about scams and tactics to get people to buy things they do not need. Encourage your loved one to be aware and get a second opinion before buying.

- SAFETY – Walk around your loved one's home and see if there might be anything that concerns you - overloaded extension cords, wobbly furniture or railings, area rugs that could be trip hazards. Take steps to ensure your loved one's home is as safe as possible.

Summary

There is no magical age when you should start to be concerned about a parent or loved one. Some people may need assistance as early as their 40's or 50's and for others, they may be self sufficient into their 80's or 90's. The point is this, be prepared, know what to look for, and be there for a loved one when he needs help. Many older adults will never ask for help as they may place their independence and privacy above all else. There can be a significant benefit to engaging in occasional conversations, and asking about his day-to-day life.

Although each of our stories is unique, there are many themes that reoccur and predominant issues that most families face. Reading this Guide and applying the information to your situation is a great first step. Also, seek support and counsel from people who have recently faced, or are facing similar life challenges. Reach out to family advisors, organizations and support groups for information and perspectives. You will quickly find that people are ready, willing and able to help and comfort you along every step of your journey. Do not hesitate to ask.

Be careful not to focus on the "here and now" without recognizing the many related issues. As our puzzle pieces suggest, each new issue and decision you face will impact other issues in the same puzzle piece, and issues in at least two other puzzle pieces. Do not focus solely on the issue at hand and get blindsided by seemingly unrelated issues.

If you have not already discovered this, you will quickly find that life is unpredictable. Regardless of where you are in the process, take time to understand the predominant issues and options. Be prepared for each new challenge.

Let me close this chapter with an excerpt from a letter I received in October 2003 that confirms the hope there is for each new day and decision you face.

> *"Many thanks for your Resource Guide and taking the time to speak with me personally. I find your information and perspectives to be quite interesting and encouraging, though a bit daunting to realize all the decision points ahead."*

Getting Started

KEY LEARNINGS – *Top three learnings from this chapter:*
1.
2.
3.

ACTION ITEMS - *Things you want to do, or do differently:*		
Check when Completed	*Action Item*	*Target Completion Date*

2

Clarity in Purpose

What is your purpose? This chapter focuses on the two primary points of view. The first viewpoint is that of the care recipient (current or future), and the second is that of the care provider, or caregiver. I suggest the framework of this chapter be the basis for all interactions between family members.

> *For professionals, whether a medical professional, attorney, financial advisor, insurance agent or other, I believe you have a responsibility to inform and educate your clients and patients so that they have the information to make informed decisions. Do not withhold information about a product or service because you do not think they are going to want it, or they are too young to consider these types of issues. Also, help people understand challenges they are likely to face, even if the issues are outside your specific area of expertise. I find attorneys offer the legal perspective, bankers and brokers offer financial advice, and doctors and nurses offer medical advice. When this happens, families may not receive basic practical advice.*

Although most people have good intentions, the care process can be challenging and good intentions are not always recognized. Remember that is it usually easier for people to give than receive. Many older adults have been self-sufficient all their lives and find it hard to accept support. Receiving requires acceptance of help that may be needed. Many older people may be concerned about being a burden to others or becoming vulnerable.

For the benefit of the care recipient and the caregiver(s), I suggest that when your family focuses on an issue, give considerable thought to what you are trying to accomplish and why. I encourage you to look beyond the quick or easy solution that will get you through the crisis, and instead take the time to identify a solution that offers a longer term benefit. Often families implement a quick fix, only to have to deal with the same issue again and again. Think about what a successful solution or arrangement might look like. In other words, if you were to look back in a month, how might you determine the success of your decision?

When talking with family members about ideas or concerns, you may find it beneficial to use "I" statements rather than "You" statements. "I" statements are less threatening and often better received. What you say and how you say it can be equally important. Remember that different is not good or bad, right or wrong, it is just different. Keep that in mind as you talk to family members and work toward solutions.

Think of a situation… buying a sweater, selecting a new car, or ordering off of a menu. The commonality is that in each of these situations you have choices. People often do not come to the same conclusions. What might be obvious to you may not be obvious to someone else. Besides your opinion; consider your parent or loved one's opinion, as it may be opposite.

If you are planning ahead, I suggest you consider how other members of your family such as aunts, uncles, and grandparents have aged. Is there a pattern of your parent's genealogy and health history that might suggest a certain medical condition or life expectancy?

For example, the longevity in Bob Hope's family, especially with his dad living to be 99 years old, was a sign that Mr. Hope was likely to live a long life. In the case of David Letterman, it was probably not a surprise when he underwent emergency quintuple heart bypass surgery in January of 2000 at the age of 52. Why? Because his family had a history of heart disease and his father died of a heart attack when in his fifties.

It should be no surprise why the life insurance industry asks applicants about the health history of their parents, as it is one of the best predictors of the health and well-being of the children. If your parent's mother and father, or brothers and sisters, have aged a certain way, your parent is more likely than not, to age in a similar fashion. I know for my mother's side of the family, cancer was a concern and neither grandparent had lived past their early 70's. This held true for their children – my mom and her siblings. On my father's side, his relatives tended to live until their late 70's and early 80's. The same held true for my father.

Clarity In Purpose

Diagnosis vs. Prognosis

At whatever time you learn of a medical concern, it is important to recognize that a 'Diagnosis' and 'Prognosis' are two different things. People that focus on the diagnosis find they are taking a medical focus. Their purpose becomes understanding the illness or disease. People that focus on the Prognosis focus on the person.

The 'Diagnosis' has to do with identifying a medical condition by its symptoms and places a name or label on a person's condition. For example, "Mrs. Smith is showing early stages of Alzheimer's."

The 'Prognosis' has to do with the prospect of recovery and the anticipated progression of the diagnosed condition. In other words, what can be expected or how will the condition become apparent in a person's life? How will it impact a loved one's functioning (mental and physical) and care requirements?

The following are examples of medical conditions commonly diagnosed from a person's symptoms:

- Chronic debilitating disease (i.e., Alzheimer's, Parkinson's, Arthritis, Osteoporosis)
- Life-threatening illness (i.e., Cancer, Heart condition)
- Medical concern (i.e. High-Risk Pregnancy, High Cholesterol)
- Injury, Illness or Surgery (i.e. Broken Hip, Diabetes, Pneumonia)

When a medical diagnosis is made, a common reaction is for people to search the Internet for information to become familiar with the illness or disease. Use the Internet with caution! A friend once made a profound statement that seems worth repeating. When a parent is diagnosed with a disease, *"there should be a mandatory 30 day waiting period before anyone is allowed to go to the Internet to look for information about the disease."* Why? Because the average person will find more information than they can ever comprehend and, all too often, the worst possible scenarios are presented. As such, people begin to *"flip out."* Then they start to question *"why didn't my parent's doctor tell me of all this?"* So, proceed with caution and do not try to become an expert overnight. Also, if you turn to the Internet for information, search multiple sites. There is good information and junk on the Internet. I simply suggest that the *"buyer beware."*

People are often overwhelmed when they are informed of a medical diagnosis, regardless of whether it was unexpected or there were indications. The individual, their family and friends often find themselves having to face new realities and the associated challenges ahead. Common concerns include: *What to do? How to help? What to expect? Who to call? What expenses are covered by private or public (Medicare) insurance?*

Understanding the prognosis will help you give consideration to the limitations a person is likely to encounter and the type of support a loved one may need. If you understand how a medical condition is likely to impact a person's life, then your purpose becomes much clearer and you will have an easier time anticipating challenges and acting to help loved ones. You will want to consider how a diagnosed medical condition will impact the following:

- Physical strength and coordination
- Mobility and reflexes
- Hearing and vision
- Mental capacity and memory
- Logic, judgment and reasoning
- Decision making capability
- Anxiety and activity levels
- Ability to focus on a particular activity
- Ability to care for self
- Ability to take medicines as directed
- Ability to handle personal affairs
- Ability to live independently

Understanding the limitations a person is likely to face is essential to provide the appropriate care and support.

Progression of a Medical Condition (Typical Scenarios)

The graphs below illustrate three typical scenarios of progression for a medical condition. The horizontal axis represents <u>Time</u> and the vertical axis represents <u>Severity</u>. These scenarios may make it easier to imagine and discuss with others how a loved one's needs may change.

40

PROGRESSION: Gradual progression of a medical condition over time (example: Alzheimer's, Arthritis, Diabetes).

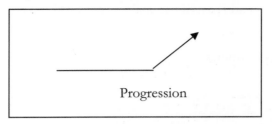

SUDDEN ONSET WITH PROGRESSION: Sudden onset (example: Stroke, Heart failure, Kidney failure) with progression over time.

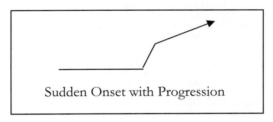

SUDDEN ONSET, EXPECTED RECOVERY: Sudden onset (example: Broken Hip, Pneumonia), however, with the proper medical treatment, the person is expected to make a full recovery.

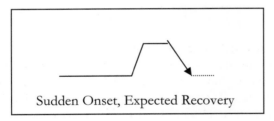

Regardless of the scenario, as a medical condition progresses, limitations may appear in many different ways. It is important for family and friends to have an understanding of a loved one's care requirements and the changes that are likely to occur.

At such time as your loved one is diagnosed with a medical condition, consult your physician and other medical professionals for information and advice specific to your situation. Also, contact the appropriate national organizations for information and to learn about resources and support services that might be available in your area. To help you get started, a partial list of national organizations follows.

National Organizations

Organization	Website Address	Telephone Number
Alzheimer's Association	www.alz.org	800-272-3900
American Cancer Society	www.cancer.org	800-227-2345
American Diabetes Association	www.diabetes.org	800-342-2383
American Heart Association	www.americanheart.org	800-242-8721
American Stroke Association	www.strokeassociation.org	888-478-7653
Arthritis Foundation	www.arthritis.org	800-283-7800
Leukemia & Lymphoma Society	www.leukemia.org	800-955-4572
National Mental Health Association	www.nmha.org	800/969-6642
National Osteoporosis Foundation	www.nof.org	202-223-2226
Parkinson's Disease Foundation	www.pdf.org	800-457-6676

The Care Recipient's Perspective

The care recipient's perspective can be challenging for family and friends to recognize and appreciate. To help you understand the care recipient's perspective, I recommend watching the movie On Golden Pond. There are some wonderful scenes where Mr. Thayer offers a glimpse into his world, his fears and his frustrations.

Give consideration to what may be going through the mind of loved one's who are aging, ill or injured. They may be scared about diminishing mental and physical abilities, be concerned about being a burden to family, or be fearful of dying. A person may prefer to ignore the facts, be unwilling to admit they are part of 'a class' (e.g. senior citizens), or may fear losing their independence. Many older adults that have lived through the Great Depression may fear spending money or be concerned about depleting their life savings. People may also fear the future or fear loneliness. The list goes on and on. When you try to figure out why a person acts and does things, think about what might be going through their minds. Talk and ask questions.

When a loved one is diagnosed with a medical condition or is suddenly hospitalized, there are several natural reactions that are common to people taking on the role of family caregiver. I share these scenarios to help you understand the care recipient's viewpoint.

NATURAL REACTION #1: *"What Am I Going To Do?"*

When a loved one faces a crisis situation, it is common for a family caregiver's response to be *"What am I going to do?"* I suggest that before 'you' do anything, you should put yourself in the shoes of the person who is facing a challenge(s). Many schools that offer courses on Gerontology, conduct exercises with their classes to help students better appreciate the realities many older adults face. From putting tape over a person's glasses so they do not see as clearly, to restricting one's legs so they are forced to shuffle, people quickly come to appreciate the limitations loved ones may face.

NATURAL REACTION #2: *Treat People Differently*

When a loved one faces a challenge or is labeled with a medical condition, family and friends have a tendency to treat the person differently. I suggest that you treat the person the same as before a medical condition existed. Instead, what you should treat differently is the circumstances. Let me say that again, do not treat the person differently, treat the circumstances differently. When I talk about the circumstances, I am focusing on the environment as opposed to the person. For example, say a person is experiencing hearing loss. Treat the person with the same loving kindness as before. To address the circumstance of hearing loss, you might reduce background noises, speak slower and louder, and enunciate your words more clearly. If a person has dementia, it is important to treat the circumstances differently to help reduce potential anxiety, agitation or confusion. In so doing, you would not want to put your loved one on the spot, asking her a complex question, or put her in a situation where she may be over stimulated.

NATURAL REACTION #3: *"Let Me Do That"*

When a person faces a limitation, regardless if the situation is a result of age, illness or injury, a natural tendency for family and friends is to overcompensate for the person. I call this the *"Let Me"* mentality. Someone faces some sort of limitation and people jump in offering to do it for them… "*Let me do that.*" Although your gestures may seem like the right thing to do, they are often unnecessary and even demoralizing. One frequently asked question I receive is: "*Why do you think so many older people resist assistance from family members?*" Many people think the answer is that older people can be stubborn or set in their ways. I have a different philosophy. My guess is that people are hesitant to place themselves in a situation where they become vulnerable. For example, if a loved one accepts a family member's assistance with one activity, how is he going to be able to say 'NO' the next time a son or daughter offers to help? In other words, I would rather not accept any help, as opposed to having someone come in, take over and start doing things their way.

The movie <u>Driving Miss Daisy</u> clearly portrays the 'Let Me' concept. Dan Ackroyd hires Morgan Freeman and tells him that his mother cannot fire him. Then, as Dan Ackroyd explains to Jessica Tandy that he hired Morgan Freeman, she says: "*Last I knew I had rights…..*" People do not want to be treated differently because they are old or infirmed. People want to be treated for who they are, not for what they have or have lost. I believe that all people, regardless of age have a basic wish to feel needed and appreciated. If a person loses his or her purpose, I often see what is referred to as a 'Failure to Thrive.' In other words, what's the purpose of living any more? People may simply avoid situations or give up entirely.

Transitioning to Retirement

Many older people who have worked their entire life have a challenging time transitioning from work life into a life of retirement. Imagine using skills and abilities on a daily basis and then suddenly stopping. Whether a person worked in a factory or was responsible for directing a team of people, everyone likes to feel as though his or her contributions are important and valuable. When a person retires and a business continues to operate without them, people often question their value.

As a result of a sudden change in one's work life, it is critically important to fill one's time with activities of purpose. Volunteer work, hobbies or other activities can give a person a reason to wake up in the morning. Also think what it must be like earning an income all your life and then suddenly the income stops. It can often be difficult for retirees to make the switch from earning and saving to spending. The point is that care recipients often internalize challenges that family members never recognize or acknowledge.

The Caregiver Perspective

When a loved one is diagnosed with a medical condition, is hospitalized or finds himself facing challenges, family members and friends are often the ones to drop everything and come to one's aid. While it seems that everyone has jam-packed schedules, it is amazing how health related issues can instantaneously get people to reprioritize everything at a moments notice.

When taking on the role of caregiver, you will quickly find yourself dealing with issues you never before expected. Taking on the role of family caregiver can be difficult. Moreover, many family members do not view themselves as a 'caregiver.' Determining when a person crosses the line between being a concerned, loving family member to family caregiver can be challenging. This is especially true for people who start off doing an occasional task and find their responsibility grows over time. I believe that it is important for you to recognize yourself as a caregiver for one primary reason. Once someone declares that they are a caregiver, I find that the person is more likely to seek information, such as this book, and reach out in the community for support and direction.

So what is the role of a caregiver? I believe that caregivers should support, encourage and love the care recipient. Stated another way; follow the Golden Rule, *"Do unto others as you would have them do unto you."* Okay, that may seem rather vague to many of you, so let me expand on that. Caregivers provide what I refer to as TLC. When I speak of TLC, most people think of the obvious Tender Loving Care. Additionally, I like to remind people of the importance of Touch, Listen and Coach.

- TOUCH. When words can not express your feelings or concerns, the best thing may simply be to put your arm around a loved one or hold her hand. Sometimes just being there is all a person wants to needs.

- LISTEN. I'm sure you have heard the saying that people have two ears and only one mouth for a purpose. Let your loved ones express her feeling and fears. Avoid the tendency to jump in, take charge and 'fix it.'

- COACH. It can help for caregivers to offer perspectives or different points of view to help a care recipient determine what might be the best. Pride often gets in the way of people's choices. People needing care do not want to impose or be a burden on their family and friends. Caregivers should constantly reinforce that '*It's Okay*,' whatever the circumstances. Help your loved one not to feel ashamed or embarrassed. Whether he is having trouble maneuvering the steps, cannot turn a door handle, wets himself on occasion or anything else, it is important to reinforce that "*It's Okay*", while coaching him so that he can avoid future situations or struggles.

How Do I Best Help?

Have reasonable expectations of yourself and other people that are involved. Do not expect too much, too quick. Celebrate each small success. Realize that often times the more people try to help, the more they are rejected and criticized. For care recipients, rejection may be a coping mechanism that often serves to create attention. For some people, negative attention through conflict can be better than no attention at all. Also, do not try to force your opinion on someone else. Make your point and convey why you are suggesting what you are suggesting.

If you want to help but a loved one expresses he does not want your help, maybe you start helping anyway. Many older people who have been self-sufficient for their entire adult lives may not know how to accept assistance. While a person may express that he does not want assistance, if he starts to receive assistance, he might find he likes the extra help.

There can be a fine line between helping too much and not enough. Ideally, family members should think about how they can encourage loved ones. Develop and implement a plan that meets the physical, social and psychological needs of the care recipient. The two types of care plans are: '*Habilitative*' and '*Rehabilitative*.'

- '*Habilitative*' care is appropriate in situations where a person is expected to gradually lose the ability to provide self-care and live independently. Since a person's dependence is expected to increase over time, the goal of a 'Habilitative' care plan is to help the person to function at their highest possible level.

- *'Rehabilitative'* care is appropriate in situations where a person is expected to make a full or partial recovery. Since a person's dependence is expected to be temporary, the focus of a 'Rehabilitative' care plan is to assist and encourage people to relearn or regain skills with the goal of restoring independence.

Besides wanting a person to maintain skills and abilities, I encourage you and your family to place 'Dignity' at the top of your list. The concepts behind Dignity are twofold. Internal and External.

First it is critical for your loved one to feel as though he is important and to have an internal feeling of love and worth. Importance suggests that the care recipient matters and that he has the right to make decisions for himself. It does not matter how honorable the intentions of family members and friends might be, if the person you are trying to help is resistant. As long as the care recipient is competent to make decisions, he has the final say – whether you agree or disagree. Second, is the concept of respectability or external appearance. Respectability has to do with the presentation of a person – how he outwardly appears to others (e.g., appearance, smell). External dignity issues include such things as:

- Incontinence – ability to control one's bladder and bowels
- Mobility – getting around (e.g. walking, cane, wheelchair, etc)
- Dental care – brushing teeth and caring for dentures
- Eye glasses – keeping the lenses clean and prescriptions up-to-date
- Grooming – washing hair, brushing hair, shaving
- Appearance and cleanliness of clothing

Having talked to hundreds and hundreds of people over the years, I have found that care recipients simply want to look respectable, feel valued and not be forgotten.

Heart and Hand Issues

As suggested with the explanations of TLC above, TLC issues are centered mainly on the Heart and feelings. Hand issues, which are often easier for people to grasp, are more task-oriented.

It is not uncommon for older people to find they need some assistance with basic tasks. A person who is ill or injured may also have physical needs. Needs are often referred to as Activities of Daily Living (ADL). As the name suggests 'Activities of Daily Living' are those things which people engage in on a daily basis. These activities are basic to caring for one's self and maintaining independence. ADL's are classified into two distinct areas: personal care (ADL's) and independent living (IADL's). Although both are critically important, there is a tendency for people to focus on the aspects of personal care.

- **Activities of daily living** are daily personal care activities such as bathing (sponge, bath or shower), getting dressed, getting in or out of bed or a chair (also called transferring), using the toilet, eating, and getting around or walking.

- **Instrumental activities of daily living** are activities about independent living and include preparing meals, managing money (writing checks, paying bills), shopping for groceries or personal items, maintaining a residence/performing housework (e.g. laundry, cleaning), taking medications, using a telephone, handling mail, and traveling via way of car or public transportation.

Physical or mental limitations may restrict a person's ability to perform activities of daily living. When a person has a limitation, he has an inability to independently perform one or more daily living activities. A three-part scale is often used to determine dependence or deficit for each activity.

INDEPENDENT ↔ ASSISTANCE NEEDED ↔ DEPENDENT

- INDEPENDENT suggests a person can perform tasks without assistance.

- ASSISTANCE NEEDED suggests a person can perform tasks with assistance from a human being, support device or both.

- DEPENDENT suggest a person is unable to perform tasks on his own.

Why is it important to be aware of a person's limitations with 'Activities of Daily Living'?

- Recognizing a person's limitations is the first step to develop a care plan to provide the appropriate type and level of assistance.

- Determining the type of ADL care that is needed enables families to assign caregiver roles and become educated on how to perform ADL care appropriately to meet the unique needs of a loved one.

- Admission policies for Adult Day services, care communities and institutions often reflect ADL's to determine eligibility and placement for a certain type of care.

- Long-term care insurance policies often rely on ADL measures (the inability to perform certain ADL's) to determine whether an individual qualifies for benefits.

Caregiver Concerns

People taking on the caregiver role often find themselves in unexpected and unfamiliar situations. Also, there is a tendency for the caregivers' health to suffer as they provide care for a loved one. Caregiver burnout is a real concern that many people overlook. The Alzheimer's Association suggests the following <u>10 Warning Signs of Caregiver Stress</u>:

1.) Denial about the disease and its effects on the person who has been diagnosed – *"I know mom is going to get better."*

2.) Anger at the person with Alzheimer's. – *"If he asks me that question one more time, I'll scream."*

3.) Social Withdrawal from friends and activities – *"I don't care about getting together…anymore."*

4.) Anxiety about facing another day and what the future holds – *"What happens when he needs more care than I can provide?"*

5.) Depression begins to affect the ability to cope – *"I don't care anymore."*

6.) Exhaustion makes it nearly impossible to complete necessary daily tasks – *"I'm too tired for this."*

7.) Sleeplessness caused by a never ending list of concerns – *"What if she wanders out of the house or falls and hurts herself?"*

8.) Irritability leads to moodiness and triggers negative responses and reactions – *"Leave me alone."*

9.) Lack of Concentration makes it difficult to perform familiar tasks – *"I was so busy, I forgot we had an appointment."*

10.) Health Problems begin to take their toll, both mentally and physically – *"I can't remember the last time I felt good."*

Ways to reduce Caregiver Stress

- Become educated about the illness or ailment and how it is likely to impact a person.

- Learn about caregiving and helpful techniques.

- Seek assistance from family, friends, and community resources.

- Take care of yourself, eat right, exercise and get plenty of rest.

- Accept changes as they occur.

- Be realistic about what you can do.

- Keep a journal and express yourself on paper.

- Give yourself credit for what you have accomplished; do not feel guilty if you lose your patience or cannot do everything on your own.

A Caregiver's Bill of Rights

Caregivers often find it difficult to maintain their physical and emotional health while caring for a loved one. A Caregiver Bill of Rights was developed years ago to help caregivers recognize their responsibilities and limitations. There are many different versions of The Caregiver's Bill of Rights which is believed to have first been published by the AARP. The version that follows is attributed to the Cincinnati Catholic Social Services Caregiver Assistance Network (www.cssdoorway.org).

1. I have the right to take care of myself. This is not an act of selfishness. It will give me the capability of taking better care of my care receiver.

2. I have the right to occasionally get angry, be depressed, and express other difficult feelings.

3. I have the right to reject attempts by my care receiver (either conscious or unconscious) to manipulate me through guilt, and or depression.

4. I have the right to take pride in what I am doing and to applaud the courage it sometimes takes to meet the needs of the person I am caring for.

5. I have the right to appreciation and emotional support for my decision to accept the challenge of providing care.

6. I have the right to protect my assets and financial future without severing my relationship with the care receiver.

7. I have the right to respite care during emergencies and to care for my own health, spirit and relationships.

8. I have the right to provide care at home as long as physically, financially and emotionally feasible; however, when it is no longer feasible, I am obligated to explore other alternatives, such as a residential care community.

9. I have the right to maintain facets of my own life that do not include the person I care for, just as I would if he or she were healthy. I know that I do everything that I reasonably can for this person, and I have the right to do some things just for myself.

10. I have the right to protect my individuality and my right to make a life for myself that will sustain me when my care receiver no longer needs my help.

11. I have the right to seek help from others even though my care receiver may object. I recognize the limits of my own endurance and strength.

12. I have the right to expect all family members, men and women, to participate in the care of aging relatives.

13. I have the right to receive consideration, affection, forgiveness, and acceptance for what I do for my loved one for as long as I offer these qualities in return.

14. I have the right to temporarily change my living environment as needed to aid in caring for aging care recipients.

15. I have the right to expect professionals, in their area of specialization, to recognize the importance of palliative care and to be knowledgeable about the concerns and options related to older people and caregivers.

16. I have the right to sensitive, supportive responses by employers in dealing with unexpected or severe care needs.

17. I have the right to receive training in caregiving skills, along with accurate understandable information about the condition and needs of the care recipient.

18. I have the right to expect and demand that as new strides are made in finding resources to aid physically and mentally impaired persons in our country, similar strides will be made toward aiding and supporting caregivers.

It is important for caregivers to realize his or her own limitations to maintain a healthy attitude and not feel guilty if he or she is not able to do everything.

Developing a Care Plan

Understanding a loved one's 'Diagnosis' and 'Prognosis,' and being familiar with their current limitations are the first steps to developing a plan. The next steps involve determining the 'What', 'Who' and 'How' of the care plan. Questions to consider include:

- What specific care or assistance is needed and anticipated?

- Who in the family will share the caregiving responsibility, and who will take on the primary role?

- What is the availability of family members to serve as caregivers, and do they have special skills or training that could help?

- What are the designated tasks and responsibilities for each person?

My sister and I divided the responsibilities for the care of our parents. I took the lead for our dad and she took the lead for our mom. This way, we were better able to address any male/female concerns. My sister also handled scheduling medical appointments and made most healthcare decisions. I took the lead handling personal, financial and legal matters.

Give some thought to the responsibilities for your situation and who can provide the needed assistance. If you find yourself in a situation where it seems like you are doing all the work, and none of the responsibilities are being shared by your siblings, ask for assistance. Quite often siblings have no idea how much time and effort someone is spending providing care and support. If this is the case with your family, I encourage you to create a list of all the things you do on a weekly basis and share it with your family. Indicate things that you need help with, point out responsibilities that do not require physical presence, and ask for help.

In situations where your family is unable to provide the needed physical care, make sure you understand the care options that might be available in your area, and decide which option(s) is best for your situation.

Clarity In Purpose

Regardless of whether care is provided by a family member, friend or care professional, it is important to keep perspective on the following five "P's":

PURPOSE: A natural reaction of caregivers is to over-care for a loved one. A good slogan to keep in mind is to "*Help only when help is needed.*" When considering how to help, think of what you are trying to accomplish and why.

PACE: Everyday tasks can be overwhelming to a person with limitations. Breaking a task into small parts can make things simpler. Also, having several milestones provides opportunities for more frequent celebrations or feelings of achievement.

PROMPT: Give encouragement and direction that enables a person to complete the task on his own. Caregivers should resist completing a task on a loved one's behalf, even though she might complete the task more easily and quickly.

PROVIDE: Provide assistive devices as appropriate that enable a loved one to maintain his mobility (such as a cane, walker, or wheelchair) and independence (use of hearing and vision aids, dentures, and other adaptive devices).

PRESERVE: Always provide care in a manner that preserves a person's dignity. The frustration and humiliation people often face as a result of losing ability, and being dependent on others, can be discouraging. Allowing choice and participation in one's own care helps maintains a loved one's dignity.

If your care plan involves providing physical assistance, be sure you know how to do so safely. There are specific techniques for helping people transfer from a bed to a chair, helping a person up from the toilet, assisting someone in and out of a bathtub or in and out of a car. To prevent injury to yourself, seek training and assistance to learn the various techniques.

When to Publicly Acknowledge a Condition?

People are generally reluctant to make public any type of personal medical challenge. Michael J. Fox and Charlton Heston appear to be more of the exception than the rule. Many people never go public as they do not want to admit they have a medical condition. Others may not go public because they fear they will be treated differently. People want to be defined by their personality, not by a disease. For example, in the workplace employees want to be treated based on their capabilities and performance, not their diagnosis. Some people are embarrassed about a condition and may be afraid others will start talking behind their back. What is interesting is that in recent years many people have come forward.

The Wall Street Journal featured an article (August 22, 2002) entitled <u>Another Agony of Alzheimer's: Deciding How – and When – to Say: "I Have It.'</u> In the article Jeffery Zaslow wrote, *"Every day on average, 986 Americans are diagnosed with Alzheimer's …steals your lucidity, thought by thought… Most families and patients have suffered silently until the symptoms were too conspicuous for others to ignore. So what are some benefits to speaking up? If you're not hiding your illness, you'll feel less stress when you forget someone's name or do something odd. Also, you can seek support, and your loved ones can make better use of community resources. If you don't go public there is often needless isolation out of fear."*

The article also told the story of a lady and her personal experience. *"At first, I didn't want to tell anyone, she says. Only her husband knew…Four months later, when they dropped the Christmas cards in the mailbox, it was both terrifying and a relief."* In the cards, she wrote: *"I have it, I can't deny it, and I will die of it eventually, but the more people hear about it, the less scary it gets."*

Elder Abuse

As I conclude this chapter on purpose, let me share some important information on elder abuse. Elder abuse is a real problem on which we can not turn our backs. It is estimated that 1 in 20 older adults is abused each year, and that number is expected to rise. Only one in eight cases is believed to be reported. Abused elderly people rarely tell or report the abuse because of shame or embarrassment, family loyalty, fear of retaliation, resignation or powerlessness, lack of credibility, or fear of placement into a nursing home or institution.

Elder Abuse includes physical abuse, psychological abuse, exploitation and neglect.

- Physical abuse is non-accidental bodily harm, and can be identified by cuts, bruises, burns, confinement, isolation and change in behavior

- Psychological abuse is deliberate conduct that causes mental anguish to a person such as yelling and putting people down.

- Exploitation has to do with theft or misuse of money, assets or other valuables.

- Neglect is indicated by daily living needs that are not being met by the caregiver or the older adult. Neglect may involve lack of personal hygiene, dirty or unsanitary living environment, inadequate health care, etc.

Elder Abuse is everyone's business. If you suspect a person is being abused, contact Adult Protective Services or your local authorities. Every caregiver should love and honor the elderly and infirmed, not to neglect and abuse them.

Summary

As a caregiver, make sure to give consideration to the care recipient's perspective and feelings. Likewise, if you are a care recipient, give consideration to the caregiver's role. Realize that most people try the do their best and that most everyone has good intentions. It is often how those intentions are communicated or demonstrate that can be challenging. Take the time to watch the movies On Golden Pond and Driving Miss Daisy, and realize you are not the first person to encounter challenges associated with aging or illness. Reach out to others for support, direction and encouragement.

Dealing with an older parent can be extremely challenging. This challenge is often magnified because family members usually have no idea how a parent is going to react to an expressed concern over his well-being and attempts to help him. Also, role reversal can be difficult to accept. After all, your parent took care of you all her life, now you are asking her to take on the child role so you can parent her. This can be a tough pill to swallow. Here are a few words of advice:

1. Be honest and appropriately straight-forward.
2. Make the care recipient's safety and the safety of those around him or her of critical importance. Also, realize that your goal of safety may be opposite to your parent's goal of independence.
3. If you have siblings, make sure everyone is in agreement on the issues and roles.
4. Talk to your parent in a non-threatening manner.

5. Do not try to force change overnight. Take your time and accept small victories.

6. Do not force your beliefs or wishes on your parent.

A popular saying in the long-term care industry is: *"One parent can raise several children; however, several children can not take care of a parent."* The point is that being a caregiver can be difficult. Take care of yourself. Recognize your limitations and find strength in others who have been down the road before. If you do not take care of yourself and you find yourself getting run down, you will not be in a position to provide care to your loved one.

While I touched on the reality of elder abuse, recognize that an illness may make a person belligerent or angry causing the caregiver to catch the brunt of the abuse. Take it in stride, knowing that your loved one may not be of sound mind and ability.

KEY LEARNINGS – *Top three learnings from this chapter:*
1.
2.
3.

ACTION ITEMS - *Things you want to do, or do differently:*		
Check when Completed	*Action Item*	*Target Completion Date*

Lifestyle Planning

The first two chapters laid important ground work, and hopefully have helped to put aging and caregiving into perspective. In this chapter, I introduce the Lifestyle puzzle piece, discuss medical conditions, alternatives to understand one's functioning level and share select community services. Often it is a hospitalization, fall, medical diagnosis or other crisis situation that causes a family to recognize that a loved one may have needs. Chapters 4, 5 and 6 are also dedicated to Lifestyle issues. Because of the complexity and variety of alternatives, a chapter is dedicated to each of the following topics:

- Transportation Concerns
- Living Environments
- Care Options

So, something just is not right, but you are not sure what it is, or what to do. You have worked through the 10 Considerations in Chapter #1 and you know it is time to get more involved in a loved one's life. Deep down inside you feel as though something can be done to help a loved one.

According to the Florida Mental Health Institute, *"The current generation of American seniors does not seek care as often as needed, so it takes resources to reach out and educate them, experts say. Depression, dementia and substance abuse account for the majority of the mental health issues among the elderly. Depressed elders use three times as much health care, and incur two times the health care costs as non-depressed elders. They make seven times the number of emergency room visits; have three times as many deaths after a heart attack and nearly three times the incidents of stroke."* (Source: <u>Seniors' mental problems often untreated</u>, Cincinnati Business Courier – 6/20/03)

According to Hanley-Hazelman, a treatment center for chemical dependency in West Palm Beach, Florida, alcohol is a problem for an estimated 8 million older Americans. *"People just don't connect sweet little gray-haired grandmothers with alcoholism, according to the centers director of older adult services. Many people use alcohol and/or sedatives to relieve pain, grief or depression. For many who begin to drink later in life, "the biggest problem is that they have lost a sense of purpose. They don't feel needed anymore,"* according to the Center's Director. (Source: <u>Addictions tarnish the golden years</u>, by Georgia Tasker – Knight Rider News Service, The Cincinnati Enquirer – 11-12-03)

A Senior Moment? Maybe

While most of us have probably lost our keys or misplaced something that was under our nose the whole time, a frequent question people have is, *"Is there a reason to be concerned, or might it just be a Senior Moment?"* If a loved one appears to have lost interest in things he once enjoyed, or if a person consistently relies on someone else to make decisions, there may be a reason to be concerned.

Often people make statements such as *"Dad's going nuts,"* or *"Mom's lost her mind,"* and don't recognize treatments may be available to help a loved one. It is important to recognize and address behavioral changes when a loved one just doesn't seem right. Seek medical attention and find out what treatments are available. The Alzheimer's Association indicates that *"As many as 10 percent of all people 65 years of age and older have Alzheimer's. As many as 50 percent of all people 85 and older have the disease."*

Dementia, depression and delirium are conditions that often go undiagnosed and untreated. The incidence of all three conditions increase as people age. The challenge is to identify abnormal behavior and to decide when to pursue medical attention. While dementia, depression and delirium are all separate and unique conditions, there are many similarities. Most importantly, the treatments for each can be different. It is important to report any and all symptoms to help medical professionals, determine the cause, and make a diagnosis, so a person can receive appropriate treatment.

Let me briefly talk about these three 'D's' before I talk about the importance of getting a full medical check-up.

DEMENTIA describes disorders that affect the functioning of one's brain, and is characterized by mental decline and impairment. Dementia is generally progressive and interferes with normal daily activity. The onset is usually slow, over a period of months or years.

Dementia and Alzheimer's are two different conditions. Alzheimer's, a degenerative disorder of the brain, is reported to be the most common cause of dementia in older adults. People with Alzheimer's have dementia; however people with dementia don't necessarily have Alzheimer's. For example, people with chronic conditions such as Parkinson's can have dementia. A common form of dementia is a condition referred to as Multi-Infarct, where blood flow is cut off from a certain part of the brain (mini-stroke) resulting in permanent damage and associated loss of mental capacity.

A person with dementia often has trouble with her ability to recall information, problem solve and speak. People also may act strangely or seem moody. People with dementia often lose the ability to perform daily tasks needed to living independently. Another characteristic is an inability to make decisions or respond to questions. As a result, it is not uncommon for a person with dementia to say things like *"that's fine with me,"* or *"I'll have what you're having,"* as she can be unable to process things on her own.

- Causes: A cause of dementia is often a stroke or series of strokes in the blood vessels in the brain. For Alzheimer's or Parkinson's disease, aside from hereditary disposition, the causes are not yet known. Research is constantly providing new insight and information.

- Symptoms: Inability to use judgment and make decisions, becoming forgetful, getting lost in familiar surroundings, difficulty learning and remembering new information, withdrawing from social activities, difficultly expressing himself.

- Treatment: Several treatments may work to help people maintain their mental capacity longer. Medications that thin the blood are often administered to reduce the risk of a stroke. Medications such as Aricept®, Reminyl®, and Exelon® may be prescribed to help treat the symptoms of mild to moderate Alzheimer's. These medications essentially work to slow down the symptoms of Alzheimer's.

- Other: As conditions worsen, paranoia, delusions and hallucinations are common.

Alzheimer's is known to progress in stages. A person in the first stage will experience mild cognitive impairment that is most likely to involve memory loss. Other than memory loss, people tend to function normally. As Alzheimer's progress to the second stage, people will experience additional challenges, such as forgetting simple words, knowing how to perform once familiar tasks, and getting lost in familiar surroundings.

People with dementia, may experience other behavioral changes including Sundowning and Shadowing.

- SUNDOWNING behavior is often apparent in the late afternoon and evening. A loved one may become demanding, suspicious, upset or disoriented, see or hear things that are not there and believe things that are not true. He may pace or wander around the house when others are sleeping. Sundowning is believed to be connected to change in lighting. Also, people may be restless and tired at the end of the day and less able to cope with stress.

- SHADOWING is where a person follows or mimics the caregiver, or talks, interrupts and asks questions repeatedly. A person may become upset and agitated if caregiver wants to be alone.

DEPRESSION is a mood disorder that can affect a person's mind and body. Although many people never seek treatment for depression, those that do often experience improvement. While everyone occasionally feels depressed or sad, depression is characterized by intense sadness that lasts for a period of two weeks or longer, and impacts a person's ability to lead a normal life.

- Causes: Hereditary predisposition, physical limitations, grief or loss of a spouse or loved one, conflict, abuse, significant change in one's life, diagnosis of a medical condition, substance abuse, loneliness, reaction to medication and more.

- Symptoms: Sadness, lack of energy, feeling of hopelessness and worthlessness; changes in sleep patterns, constant aches and pains, change in appetite, difficulty concentrating and more.

- Treatment: The most common treatments include a combination of psychotherapy (talking about, identifying and addressing potential underlying life situations) and medications such as antidepressants.

- Other: Depression that goes untreated can lead to medical complications and even suicide.

Lifestyle Planning

Depression can also be the result of a chronic pain. According to an article from the May 9, 2002 edition of The Wall Street Journal, entitled, Taking the Aches Out of Aging, *"Pain shouldn't be an inevitable part of growing old. An estimated 20-40% of Americans age 65 and older suffer from long-term pain, but only a fraction receives treatment."* The article indicated that medical professionals are working to rename pain problems as "persistent pain," rather than "chronic pain," as the word chronic conjures up the notion that nothing can be done to relieve the pain. Many pain conditions can be successfully treated; improving one's functioning and decreasing pain. If you think pain may be a concern, visit the AGS Foundation website for additional information: www.HealthInAging.org/public_education/pain

If you believe someone's behavior is more than a "Senior Moment," or you sense something just isn't right, seek medical attention. Medical professionals are likely to complete a full medical work-up to identify and rule out possible causes. People who receive treatment often experience an improvement and a better quality of life.

DELIRIUM is a cognitive or mental disorder, not a disease, which appears suddenly, often within hours or days, and may come and go throughout the day. A person who is delirious appears disoriented, shows varying levels of consciousness, has disorganized speech, and an inability to comprehend what's being said. Delirium can be frightening, as a loved one acts unpredictably, is uncooperative and sometimes acts violently. It is not unusual for a delirious person to have mood swings and appear as if he is living in his own world. Also, his memory can be affected. With delirium, there is usually an underlying cause that once identified is treatable.

- Causes: Reaction to prescription medication or interaction of medications, infection, dehydration, physical illness, head injury or other trauma, substance abuse, sleep deprivation and more.

- Symptoms: Impaired thinking, unusual anxiety, and sudden personality change.

- Treatments: Once the cause is identified and treatment begins (e.g. changing medications, increasing fluids, or treating infections), there is often a quick turn-around. In situations where there may be a need to calm or sedate a person, drugs called antipsychotics may be introduced.

- Other: Physical restraints may be needed to prevent a delirious person from harming themselves or others.

Medical Considerations

Just as parents with infants and toddlers see Pediatricians specializing in adolescent care, many older people choose to see a Geriatrician or a Geriatric Nurse Practitioner (GNP). Geriatricians and GNP's receive specialized training for various complex issues specific to older adults. Their training and experience is with older patients and they may identify issues and suggest treatments differently than medical professionals not as accustom to treating seniors. If you believe a Geriatrician or GNP might be right for your situation, schedule a consultation appointment to learn more. Also, know that there are a limited number of medical professionals that specialize in geriatrics. Many specialists are already scheduling appoints three to six months out.

If you believe a care coordinator would be helpful, you might consider speaking with a Geriatric Care Manager (GCM). A GCM is a professional who specializes in helping older adults and their families with aging-related issues. GCM's often have a background in social work, as a counselor or a nurse. GCM's tend to take a more holistic or big picture approach often starting with a comprehensive assessment and development of a family care plan. With many people seeing several medical professional for different health issues, a GCM can help you coordinate aspects of care and can also help family members obtain services and support as needed. To find a Geriatric Care Manager in your area, visit www.CareManager.org.

A re-emerging specialization is physicians making house calls. Old-fashion house calls provide more personalized attention, more time with a patient and the ability for medical professional to observe one's surroundings. Many physicians are setting up 'boutique practices' where besides incurring a charge for each visit, a patient also pays a set amount annually to become one of a limited number of patients the physician accepts. Apparently, physicians making house calls are able to bill Medicare roughly 50% more than for a comparable office visit. Dr. Boling, professor of geriatrics at Virginia Commonwealth University School of Medicine estimates, *"at least two million Americans are chronically ill and homebound. House calls are especially good for patients who have limited mobility or face transportation challenges."* (Source: Wall Street Journal - 8/2/2002)

Understanding Nursing Designations

An option which was mentioned above is Geriatric Nurse Practitioners (GNP). Although GNP's are not physicians, they do have specialized training in Geriatric Medicine and care of older adults. GNP's have master degrees and are licensed to prescribe medications.

Because of all the jargon in the industry, let me take a moment to review the various nursing designations. (Source: Dept. of Labor's Occupational Outlook Handbook.)

- NURSE PRACTITIONERS have an advanced college (Master's) degree, can provide basic health care and can prescribe medicines.

- REGISTERED NURSES (RN) have an associates or bachelor's degree, or at least two years of college training.

- LICENSED PRACTICAL NURSES (LPN) have at least 9 months of technical or vocational training.)

- NURSES AIDES or Certified Nursing Assistants (CNA) have at least 75 hours of training and successful completion of a competency evaluation program.

It is difficult to know what is an appropriate ratio of nursing staff to patients, as circumstances vary tremendously. In an intensive care unit of a hospital, one nurse often cares for one patient. In a hospital ward where patients are in fairly good condition, a one-nurse-to-five-patients ratio might be excellent. When you move outside a hospital to a Nursing Home, the ratios and mix of staff are different. Check to find out what are reasonable norms in your city, investigate several options and ask questions about ratios.

Regardless of the environment and ratio, family members should always serve as extra ears and eyes to look out for a care recipient's best interests, and point out potential concerns to the medical staff. Depending on the situation, many families choose to hire a private duty nurse or companion caregiver so that a loved one is not left alone for extended periods of time.

Diseases, Ailments and Tips

When people think about aging Americans, they often associate with various diseases or ailments. Some diseases are terminal and will result in death. Others are more of a medical condition where a person lives with pain, ongoing discomfort or limitations. Ailments that are commonly associated with older adults and links to the respective organizations include:

- **Dementia / Alzheimer's** – intellectual challenges such as thinking, remembering and reasoning (www.alz.org)

- **Parkinson's** - disorder of the central nervous system, commonly seen as uncontrollable tremors or shaking (www.pdf.org)

- **Cancer** – group of many related diseases all of which involve out-of-control growth and spread of abnormal cells in any of the body's tissues (www.cancer.org)

- **Cardio Vascular Disease** – stroke, heart attack, or congestive heart failure (www.americanheart.org)

- **Huntington Disease** - degenerative brain disorder that slowly reduces an individual's ability to walk, think, talk and reason (www.hdsa.org)

- **Arthritis** - pain and stiffness in joints (www.arthritis.org)

- **Osteoporosis** - bones deteriorate and become fragile, also impacts a person's posture (www.nof.org)

How Common Are These Conditions?

- According to the Alzheimer's Association, it is estimated that 15% to 20% of people age 65 to 80 have symptoms of Alzheimer's. By the time people reach the age of 80, the frequency of symptoms increases to one in three people.

- Over 4 Million people are diagnosed with Alzheimer's disease every year, 70% of those are cared for at home.

- One million Americans including Muhammad Ali, Janet Reno, and Michael J. Fox are believed to have Parkinson's.

- One in three U.S. adults, or 69 million people have Arthritis or other chronic joint pain (Source: Chicago Caregiver Magazine – March 2003)

- Merck reports that nearly 40% of all women in their sixties have osteoporosis. And, according to the National Osteoporosis Foundation, over 2 million males and 8 million women suffer from the debilitating bone-thinning disease.

If your loved one is diagnosed with a disease, contact the national organization's local office (e.g., Alzheimer's Association) for information, resources and tips specific to the disease and to learn about support services available in your area. These organizations provide information that complements this Resource Guide. For example, besides the information on nursing home selection considerations in Chapter #5, if your loved one is diagnosed with Alzheimer's, the Alzheimer's Association suggests some other questions specific to people with dementia (Source: Special Care Unit Guidelines). For example:

- *What are the philosophy and goals of the unit to meet the special needs of persons with dementia?*

- *Ask to see the admissions and discharge criteria for the unit. Of interest may be at what point may a person with dementia has to be discharged from the unit?*

- *What is the size and design of the unit? (Certain layouts and sizes can be over stimulating for dementia residents)*

- *How is the staff selected for the unit? Is special training or education provided to those who work on the unit?*

- *How residents that wander are dealt with?*

For specific information about a medical condition and treatment options, also consult your physician or other medical professional.

Helping Families Make Life Altering Decisions

At such time as a loved one faces any type of deviation from wellness, families often struggle when trying to determine what is best. When engaging in family discussions, it is not uncommon for tension and frustrations to emerge. Many families attempt to communicate with one another, only to find themselves in conflict and in disagreement. Whether due to family dynamics or personality styles, individuals often come across as being more interested in expressing their opinions and winning others over, rather than reaching consensus and finding a workable solution to a problem. Peoples' behaviors when stressed also tend to bring out the worst outcome, at a time when everyone wants the best solution.

When this happens, we encourage you to stop and ask yourself *"Are you solving the right problem?"* To help families communicate effectively and reach agreement, I suggest you follow the step-by-step process I created that is designed to focus more on facts and less on feelings.

#1. ACCURATELY DEFINE THE ISSUE – Start your conversation by defining the issue about which you are trying to make a decision. Quite often families make the mistake of defining an issue inaccurately or too narrowly. When defining an issue, avoid 'opinion' statements as they usually suggest that there is only one acceptable outcome. For example, if you say *"Mom and dad are no longer able to live independently at home,"* the implied solution may be for mom and dad to move. If mom and dad feel strongly about remaining in their home, you are likely to meet tremendous resistance and get nowhere. Instead, define the issue as a 'question' statement. For example, ask *"Are Mom and Dad able to live independently at home, and if not, what might be some appropriate solutions?"* Asking a question suggests a willingness to discuss the situation, an openness to explore the areas of concern, consider alternatives, and not be isolated in your viewpoint.

#2. AGREE UPON THE ISSUE – Make sure everyone involved agrees on the issue before you start to address it and work toward a solution. Working toward a solution before there is issue agreement often leads to confusion and frustration as people find themselves trying to solve different problems. For example, if you embrace the opinion statement above, you would naturally focus your efforts on identifying new living environments suitable for your mom and dad. However, if you focus on the question statement, you would begin by identifying and understanding your mom and dad's limitations and needs. Agreement is also helpful in that if participants get off track, you can bring them back by re-stating the purpose of this particular discussion, and asking that other issues be tabled. If you determine that you inaccurately or too narrowly defined the issue, you can always go back to Step 1 and re-define the issue.

#3. ADDRESS THE NEEDS – When an issue is accurately defined as a question statement, families are forced to answer the question and express their viewpoints. Make sure to spend ample time talking about, and prioritizing, what is most important before jumping to conclusions. By focusing on the needs, conversations tend to be more objective and less subjective. Also, make sure to distinguish between 'needs' and 'wants' when making decisions. Needs are things that are essential to one's health, well-being and safety. Wants are things for which people have become accustomed. When families take the time to understand and address a loved one's needs, a greater number of suitable options typically emerge.

#4. ASSESS THE OPTIONS – The best way to solve a problem is to align a person's prioritized needs with the available options, to find the solution that delivers the best match. In the example above, once there is a clear understanding of the needs and what you are trying to accomplish, a logical next step would be to consider the various living environments and care options available to determine what might be best. Make sure to look at the pro's and con's of each situation and option.

#5. AGREE ON A SOLUTION – By working through steps 1 through 4, multiple solutions often emerge that families find to be suitable. Agree on the solution that appears best or is most acceptable to mom and dad. Remember, mom and dad have the ultimate say on any solution as long as they are competent.

The Decision Spectrum[SM]

The **Decision Spectrum** is a tool that I developed to help families communicate and reach decisions. While it is a simple tool, what is most important is that it works. The Decision Spectrum shows a line or continuum with two end points or extremes. Let's say you are considering living arrangements for your parent. When you begin to consider and evaluate the various arrangements, and the associated lifestyle implications, it helps to think about the situation as a spectrum of options. The spectrum shows a line or continuum with each of the end points representing an extreme position – *"Change is Needed"* and *"No Need for Change"*. In the middle, you have more a flexible position or preference – *"Change is Imminent or Preferred."*

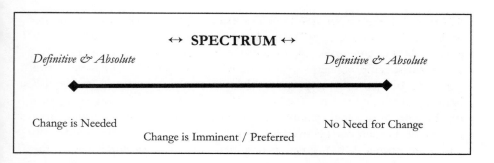

↔ **SPECTRUM** ↔

Definitive & Absolute   *Definitive & Absolute*

Change is Needed   No Need for Change
              Change is Imminent / Preferred

How to Apply the Tool

STEP 1: Take out a blank sheet of paper, draw a line across the top and show the points at each end of the spectrum relative to the issue you are addressing. Define the issue as a question statement and write it above the spectrum.

STEP 2: Make a hash mark along the continuum that represent the opinions of each family member. The hash marks are critical because they help family members visualize where everyone is along the spectrum relative to the issue being discussed. This step enables people to gain an appreciation for the concerns that will need to be confronted before any type of acceptable agreement can be reached.

> *For our family, my sister and I were at the far left extreme implying that 'Change was Needed." Our father, despite his Leukemia, was at the opposite end of the spectrum "No Need for Change". As such, we were never going to agree on living arrangements. The result? We wasted everyone's time... including our own. Our parents would agree to look at retirement communities just to make us happy...then later they would rattle off a dozen or so reasons why that community would not work for them. If we ever did agree on something, one of the parties would usually have tremendous resentment because they felt forced into something. (Note: Forced victories are false victories that create emotional burdens. This unwanted baggage often leads to deteriorating relationships.)*

> *I find that older Americans can be set in their ways. Words that people often use to characterize their aging parent include, "stubborn", "prideful" and "independent." Whatever the word is that best describes your parent, change can be hard for any of us. Coming to an agreement is often a process that takes place over time.*

STEP 3: Ask the question WHY? For example, *"Dad, why do you believe you are fine in the current situation?"* Write down the main points expressed by each person. At the same time, you'll have an opportunity to state your concerns. Focus on specific concerns you have, what you believe is important and why you believe it is important. Make sure to discuss and distinguish between needs and wants. (See below) If you find yourself at opposite ends of the spectrum, start talking about what is important and why it is important. Is each perspective true and realistic, or is someone muddled in false perceptions? Often times, people will not realize or admit something until it clearly demonstrated.

STEP 4: Consider each other's view points. Does anything that was said cause anyone to change their position? (Remember this is not about Right vs. Wrong or Winning vs. Losing) Keep in mind that a suitable solution that is acceptable to everyone may end up being somewhere in the middle of the spectrum. Throughout this process, in addition to identifying areas of concern, make sure to recognize the issues where there is agreement among family members.

STEP 5: Now that you have taken the opportunity to consider and understand other family member's points of view, go back to Step 1 and determine if the gap is narrowed and everyone is thinking more alike.

STEP 6: Assuming that the hash marks on the Decision Spectrum are clustered, start working toward specific solutions. Consider the various options that might be available, the pro's and con's of each, and work toward a solution that addresses the prioritized needs.

Needs vs. Wants

People often get so caught up and focused on what they Want, they overlook their Needs. How can you tell if something is a Need or a Want? One simple way is to listen to what someone says. For example, *"I want….."* People often focus on the things they may give up or lose when considering a change. This exercise can often help to surface fears and trepidations. Let's take a moment to clarify the distinction between Needs and Wants.

NEEDS - Things that are critically important to one's health, well being and safety. Such as:
* Floor plan/layout is conducive to one' level of mobility
* Needed services are accessible
* Cost is within one's financial means – ability to pay
* Clean environment
* Safe environment

WANTS – Things that are *"nice to have,"* often times these are things to which people have become accustomed. Such as:
* Privacy
* Inside parking
* Convenient to beauty parlor
* Convenient to places frequented
* Convenient to family members and friends

A great starting point to determine and differentiate between Needs and Wants is writing them down on paper. Once you have a list, work through the process of elimination to determine what really matters and what is reasonable to expect. When working on your list, your family may find it easier for everyone to prepare his or her own list and then compare and consolidate the lists into one master list.

If Only I Would Have…After our father passed away and my sister and I decided that a Nursing Home was best for our mother, we began making the tours and hearing the sales pitches. But we were ill-prepared. We had not discussed priorities and we found ourselves "in the moment," being influenced by things that were not important. The result? We moved our mother in and out of three different nursing homes for various reasons. The reason we decided on the third (and final) home was because we took the time to write down our needs and wants. By doing this, we were able to understand what was important and quickly move to a suitable solution. We found the perfect spot and Mom lived there for the last two years of her life. We were finally confident that we made the right decision on her behalf and had a clear understanding of what was necessary and acceptable.

Make sure your first list is general enough so you are not trying to force a solution. Also, even if something sounds obvious, write it down. Start with a general list and narrow down the alternatives.

Completing Your List

Needs and Wants lists are great for all lifestyle considerations including dietary, medication and even driving concerns. For example, say you think it is time to intervene or suggest your parent stop driving. Complete the list. You might find that your parent wants to have the autonomy and independence a car provides; however, when you get down to it, he may only drive a few times a week. Thus, the challenge may be to show that alternative methods of transportation can meet his need of going to luncheons, the barber, the doctor, drug store, the golf course, etc. Also, when giving consideration to needs, give some thought as to who else might have similar transportation needs. In other words, say your father has a weekly luncheon with someone. Maybe that person can pick-up your father, thus eliminating the need for him to drive. By identifying the needs and alternatives, people often find that many needs are much easier to address than they might think.

EXERCISE #2 – Needs vs. Wants
Create your own list of Needs and Wants on a separate piece of paper. Remember: • NEEDS are things that are critically important to one's health, well-being and safety.   • WANTS are things that are nice to have, often times these are things to which people have become accustomed.

Assessing Your Situation

One common challenge is knowing if or when a person may need and deserve assistance. While the first two chapters offered ideas and suggestions, many people want a professional opinion. This section delves more deeply into how to identify and address potential areas of concern. The questions I want to help you answer include the following:

- Is your parent or loved one functioning at a level consistent with her age and medical conditions?
- Should you be concerned about her safety, or the safety of those around her?
- Does she have impairments that require added support or care?
- Is she getting the proper nutrition, medication, etc?

Geriatric Functional Assessment

If you have concerns that your parent may not be functioning at an age-appropriate level, or if you have other concerns that may impact her safety or well being, a Geriatric Assessment or Functional Assessment can be an appropriate step. It also provides an opportunity to become more familiar with your parent's physician and begin developing a dialogue for advice, information and counsel.

Why Conduct A Functional Assessment?

1. Family members are often too close to a situation to objectively assess a loved one struggle. You may be so used to being around mom and dad that you simply do not see impairments, limitations, potential hazards, or other challenges. Loved ones may also hide or cover up things. My parents proved to be experts at masking things. By the time we realized

our parents' limitations and challenges, we were already behind the eight ball.

2. Many people simply do not know, do not want to know, or do not want to admit to themselves that their capabilities have diminished over the years. Think about it closer to home. I know many people in their 30's and 40's who are already having difficulty driving at night. Too many things going on at once can drive them crazy. They are more likely to need a nap once in a while. So, if we are already challenged in our lives, imagine the challenges an older person may be feeling.

3. People often do not understand the implications of one thing versus another. Any one task or activity in and of itself may be easy. But when you try to do a combination of five or six individual tasks that is when you have difficulty coping. What is the point? An older person can often be overwhelmed by too many things in the mix and find it difficult to cope.

4. Just as *"too many cooks spoil the broth,"* counsel from too many people can cause conflict. Take, for example, a case where an older person is seeing several doctors for many conditions. What often happens is that one doctor will prescribe a medicine; another doctor will prescribe another medicine for a different condition, and so on. A problem might be that no single doctor may be considering the interactions of the medications with each other.

5. A Functional Assessment identifies challenges your parent may be having with basic bodily functions or issues associated with leading a dignified life. Such issues include bathing, incontinence, cutting toenails, dental or denture care, hair care, and more.

The Functional Assessment is a wonderful tool to provide your parent and the family with reliable and accurate information needed to assess a situation and begin to make informed decisions. An Assessment is often a series of studies, using a variety of formats, including one-on-one conversations and interactive exercises. The Assessment can help by identifying areas where a person is functioning below the norm. It also pinpoints challenges and limitations that may hinder a person's ability to independently care for herself and function in everyday society.

Functional Assessments are usually conducted at major medical centers by a team of physicians, social workers and other healthcare professionals. Due to the time it takes to conduct an Assessment and the number of medical personnel involved, fewer and fewer medical facilities offer a comprehensive Assessment.

To find out more, speak with your parent's doctor or to find a medical center that conducts Geriatric Assessments in your area, go to: www.americangeriatrics.org. Although the specifics of an Assessment may vary by state, medical facility and doctor, a medical professional can help you determine the most appropriate solution and explain the Assessment alternatives available in your community. Keep in mind that with the combination of a decreasing number of medical professionals in the field of Geriatric Medicine, and more people seeking a Functional Assessment, it can often be months before someone can be seen for an Assessment.

Components of a Functional Assessment include:
- ✓ Review of concerns and what a family is hoping to accomplish.
- ✓ Review of patient information, medical history and family history.
- ✓ Review of medications being taken and why.
- ✓ Comprehensive medical exam, including review of bodily systems and mental health.
- ✓ Review of nutritional and sleep patterns.

Because many conditions affecting the elderly are common and expected, a Functional Assessment is a great way to determine if there are conditions that should be of concern. By identifying areas of concern, you can work with medical professionals and social workers to find solutions based on individual needs, to either improve or maintain the functional abilities and the quality of life. Common quality of life issues center on a person's mobility, grooming and personal care. Other issues may include ensuring adequate nutrition, the ability to manage money, societal and environment issues.

Another consideration is a loved one's ability to safely operate and control a motor vehicle. I discuss driving and transportation alternatives in the next chapter.

Managing Multiple Medications

As a result of aging, illness or injury, it is common for people to take several medications. According to J.W. Long in his book The Essential Guide to Chronic Illness, many seniors are taking multiple medications simultaneously. On average, older adults are taking 4 ½ pills at on time, with some people taking as many as 10 or 12. As a result of managing multiple medications prescribed by several medical professionals, older adults are three times more likely to have adverse drug interactions than younger adults.

Medications are a blessing and a curse. Although many people are healthier because of the availability of prescription drugs, as more people take more medications for more conditions, there is a far greater chance for a person to experience adverse reactions. Because of the many specialists who could be prescribing a medication, it is critically important to keep a running list of all the medications (over the counter, prescription and supplements) a person is taking including the frequency, dosage and prescribing doctor.

The list should be taken to all medical appointments and be readily available at one's home. When a medical professional asks about the medications a person is taking, invariably your loved one will not be able to recall each medication by name. Before a physician adds or changes a prescription, share your list of current medications and ask about potential interactions. Also, if emergency personnel ever have reason to come to your house, they will often look on or inside the refrigerator for a list of medications a person may be taking. Make sure to have a list of medications readily available at home.

Vision can also present challenges with medications. Pill containers are usually small and the writing on the bottle can be difficult to read. It is best not to have someone identify medications by color alone. Some people may require assistance preparing medicines so they know what to take and when.

Ideally you will want to help a loved one avoid taking multiple medicines that address the same or similar concern, ailment or pain, being over or under stimulated and introducing drugs that don't work well together.

For my mother, during the last six months of her life, she was on so many medications (at a cost of over $1,000 per month) that it was like she was *eating a three-course meal. Because so many doctors and medications were involved in her care, there came a point when the medications were not producing the desired effect. My sister and I had to make the decision to take her off her medications and re-introduce them one at a time to find out which one(s) were causing the problem. When her medications were not right, it was easy and unfortunate to see her discomfort.*

Big Picture Considerations

Beware of the many emotional challenges you are likely to encounter as you learn a loved one has a health concern that will impact his or her life. At such time as a person's capabilities or capacity is diminished, either as part of the normal aging process or as the result of an illness or disease, the reactions are often the same.

- It can often be difficult or even frustrating that she is not as quick or capable as you'd like.

- You can become overwhelmed as you realize you may need to do more to help or care for your parent.

- There is often frustration and anger wondering, *"Why my parent?"*

- Often there is disbelief, denial and even anger.

- Many people turn to prayer asking that their loved one's life be spared.

Once the realities set in, a common step is acceptance, coming to terms and determining what you can do to ensure your loved one's comfort and care. At this point, family members often turn to support groups and organizations specific to a disease or illness. This is not to suggest that everyone will experience the same emotions, rather, it is to help you understand that your feelings are normal and that you are not alone.

Depending on your relationship and your parent's medical condition or limitations, you may choose to spend more or less time with your parent. Specific to my parents, I chose to spend more time with my father, as his Leukemia did not change his mind and physical abilities. But, I found it difficult to keep up the frequency and duration of visits with my mother as her dementia advanced. Frankly it was hard for me to have my lasting memories of her in a confused and anxious state of mind. There is no right or wrong answer. I believe that is it important to preserve memories and ensure that a loved one's dignity is maintained to the end.

From an administrative standpoint, when an illness or other limitations are identified, the reality of a situation often sets in. It is important to ensure that your loved one has her affairs in order including Will, Power of Attorney, Living Will and Healthcare Durable Power of Attorney. See Chapter #7 – Legal Planning. Make sure you have the needed information, authority and relationships at whatever time it may be necessary to engage on your parent's behalf.

As a person's care needs increase, there can be tremendous effort required of the family to evaluate the circumstances, determine the most appropriate and suitable alternatives, engage professional services, handle the associated personal matters, and more. Just because arrangements are put in place, it does not mean that everything runs on autopilot. Instead, someone needs to ensure that professional and care services are being delivered in an acceptable manner on an on-going basis. If there are issues that do not meet your satisfaction, action may need to be taken to correct a situation or find a replacement or alternative solution.

Summary

It is critically important to understand what issues or conditions you are dealing with before you can begin to address a problem. Older adults are much more prone to health-related challenges. Family members should be aware of the type of limitations loved ones may be facing. Make sure to seek medical attention if something does not seem right. Also consider keeping a journal or other record of symptoms or observations that might help a physician make a diagnosis.

When applying the Decision Spectrum, don't be surprised if you and your parent are at different ends of the spectrum. Regardless of the issue, it can be challenging to realize and understand each others' perspectives and needs. It can be frustrating when things may seem so clear or obvious to you, but your parent has a different opinion. Remember to take things one day at a time and target small victories while working toward a bigger, more encompassing solution. Patience is a virtue about which we learn and are reminded. Think about the repercussion of forcing your opinion on someone else and keep in mind what is most important, the relationship or the outcome. Act accordingly.

Lifestyle Planning

KEY LEARNINGS – *Top three learnings from this chapter:*
1.
2.
3.

ACTION ITEMS - *Things you want to do, or do differently:*

Check when Completed	Action Item	Target Completion Date

4

Transportation Concerns

I purposefully title this chapter Transportation as opposed to Driving for good reason. I want to stress that there are more ways than one to get from point A to point B.

How many times have you been following an older person driving down the road and made a comment like, *"They shouldn't be driving!"* Or perhaps, you have passed an older driver on the highway that you might classify as dangerous, because of his extremely slow speed or erratic behavior behind the wheel.

I believe that many older adults deny their limitations because losing the privilege to drive is a threat to one's independence, and tends to make people feel vulnerable. Most people associate driving with freedom and as a right, as opposed to a privilege. But, driving is a privilege, and health limitations often require people to reconsider this privilege for their safety and the safety of passengers, other drivers and pedestrians.

Driving requires quick thinking and reactions, good perceptual abilities and split-second decision making. Although problems with vision may be apparent, other less obvious medical conditions may also present challenges. For example, someone with Diabetes may not know if he is depressing the brake because of numbness in his legs and feet. Arthritis can hinder one's ability to turn the steering wheel or to swerve to miss a foreign object in the street.

Before driving emerges as an area of concern, you might take time to talk with your loved one and agree on the characteristics or attributes that characterize a safe driver. By doing so, if there comes a point when you believe a loved one is unsafe, you will have the confidence to intervene. As you deem appropriate, you may ask your parent to agree to restrict his driving to certain hours and routes.

A Cause for Concern

Federal statistics show there were 19.1 million drivers age 75 and older in 2001. That number equates to about 10% of all drivers. According to the Insurance Institute for Highway Safety, elderly drivers, those age 65 and older, are more likely to be involved in fatal car accidents, and those accidents are more likely to involve multiple vehicles at intersections.

- The National Highway Traffic Safety Administration (NHTSA - Source: http://www.nhtsa.dot.gov) reports that people 70 years and older make up roughly 9% of the U.S. population. But, they account for close to 14% of all traffic fatalities and about 18% of all pedestrian deaths annually.

- Of traffic fatalities involving older drivers, 82% occurred during the daytime and 75% involved a second vehicle.

An article entitled <u>Older drivers unsafe at any speed?</u> in the February 19, 2004 edition of The Cincinnati Enquirer indicated the biggest risk to older drivers is injuring themselves due to their frailty. A study by the AAA Foundation for Traffic Safety, found that *"drivers 65 or older are nearly twice as likely to die in a crash as drivers age 55 to 64. Drivers over 85 were nearly four times as likely to die. As people grow older, drivers are more likely to cause a crash because of a lapse in perception, such as failing to yield or running a red light. Of drivers age 75 or older that were involved in an accident, 59% were due to a lapse in perception. For drivers 85 and older, perception lapses were cited in 67% of accidents."*

A few things immediately stand out:

1. Although it may be no surprise that this age group causes more traffic fatalities than any other (followed by teenage drivers), most people do not think of accidents involving pedestrians.
2. With such a high percentage of accidents occurring in the daylight and involving a second vehicle, it seems pretty clear that older drivers are not as responsive behind the wheel as younger drivers.
3. Failing to intervene when the safety of a loved one's driving is questionable may unnecessarily cause injury or death to others.

Transportation Concerns

So how do you determine if a loved one might be safe or unsafe on the road? Get in the car with your loved one and go for a drive with him. If he is driving consistent with his younger years, it may be safe to assume that everything is fine for now. But, if you go for a drive with someone, find yourself perspiring and having white knuckles from holding on tight that may be a sign that a person might not be safe.

Besides getting in the car and observing one's abilities behind the wheel of a car, people may have concern with a person's cognitive abilities, such as forgetting how to get to the beauty parlor. If you believe there might be memory related concerns, I encourage family members to talk. Often times when a family member or friend expresses concern and asks a loved one to voluntarily stop driving, he will agree to stop. By involving him in the decision making process, you may validate a concern that he has had for a while, and he may feel as though it is time to stop driving.

If your parent has moderate to severe dementia, he should not drive due to the risk of being in unpredictable or unfamiliar situations. A driver's assessment should be performed for a parent with early dementia to assess safety.

Many older people think that their driving is safe...after all; they've been driving for a long time. If you talk to a loved one about his driving, know that discussing driving can be a controversial and even explosive subject. At the same time, if you have concerns, but do not do anything, you are potentially threatening the well-being of your parent, fellow passengers, other drivers and pedestrians. Driving is one of the most significant elements of a person's independence. Think about it, if someone were to take away your license, you would relinquish your freedom and flexibility to go where you want, when you want. It is important not to underestimate your parent's perceived need to drive (even if he doesn't go out that often).

The National Institute on Aging estimates that over a half million people age 70 and older give up their keys each year. While many people voluntarily give up their keys, other people may continue to drive, as they do not recognize or admit a change in cognitive and sensory skills that may impair their ability to drive safely.

Driving Assessment

Driving is a tough topic because there are so many issues and risks associated with operating a motor vehicle. Safe driving requires excellent visual and sensory perception, and excellent reflexes. Besides issues already mentioned, there is also the unsettling image of how an older person might cope if he finds himself involved in an accident, with a flat tire, etc.

If your parent is driving, you might encourage him to have a cellular telephone with him at all times when he is away from home. You might also encourage or help him program his cellular phone with contact and emergency telephone numbers.

If your parent is still driving, occasionally get in the car with your loved one and go for a drive. As a passenger in his vehicle, you will be able to see for yourself how well he drives. While driving can be subjective, there are certain things you can assess including:

- Does he drive within the lines?
- What is his speed compared to the speed limit?
- Can he park with relative ease?
- Does he yield or take turns at a four-way stop?
- Is he in the correct lane for the direction he wishes to go? *(e.g., is he in the turn lane when turning?)*
- Is he paying attention and concentrating on the road?

To determine if your parent is doing well or not, it may be necessary to take him to a less familiar route.

The good news for many older people is that there are a variety of driving programs designed to help people understand their limitations and sharpen their skills. One popular program is the 55 Alive program offered by the AARP. The program is essentially a refresher course offering 8-hours of class room instruction and discussion. For more information contact the AARP at www.aarp.org/drive or 888-227-7669.

On January 13, 2005 the AAA announced that it has developed a new test — Roadwise Review™, a tool to Help Seniors Drive Safely Longer. According to the AAA, the interactive computer based test (available on CD-ROM) is designed to help seniors decide for themselves, or with their family, if they are capable of driving safely.

Transportation Concerns

The tool is designed to enable seniors to administer the test in the privacy of your home, with the help of a family member or friend. The AAA reports that there are eight functional capabilities that are most associated with safe driving.

The abilities tested in Roadwise Review include:
- Leg Strength and General Mobility
- Head/Neck Flexibility
- High- and Low-Contrast Visual Acuity
- Working Memory
- Visualization of Missing Information
- Visual Search
- Useful Field of View

The test is expected to highlight potential areas of concern for which people may not be aware. For more information or to obtain a copy of the Roadwise Review CD-ROM, contact your local AAA club or visit www.aaafoundation.org.

Another service that may be of interest is a Driver Ability Screening. Screenings are often conducted by occupational therapists and provide objective and comprehensive evaluation of the skills people need for driving. At the conclusion, the screener provides feedback and suggestions on what a person can do to improve his abilities and adjust the way he goes about driving. As appropriate, a screener might suggest special equipment and individual training to teach the driver to compensate for impairments.

If you pursue a Driver Ability Screening, be sure to understand the type of testing that is conducted. Some evaluations may take place over a 2-3 hour period and consists of classroom testing and behind-the-wheel testing by a licensed occupational therapist. Classroom evaluation focuses on extremity motor function, visual abilities, perception, reaction, and more. Behind the wheel evaluation focuses on maneuverability skills, residential roads, two and four lane highways, interstate, etc. Depending on the type of evaluation, the cost for driving evaluations varies from $250 to $800.

Places you might call to find out about driver assessment services in your area include:
1. State Bureau of Motor Vehicles.

2. A rehabilitation unit of a local hospital.

3. The local Alzheimer's Association.

Evaluations are occasionally ordered by a medical professional to assess a person's ability to resume or continue driving. Medical professionals can be a great source of information and advice on driving. If you wish to talk with your parent's physician about a driving concern, consent will be required. Federal regulations in the medical industry, namely HIPAA – the Health Insurance Portability and Accountability Act of 1996, make it against the law to discuss health related matters with anyone except the patient without written consent.

If there is a reason for concern, a physician can send a form to the State Bureau of Motor Vehicles requesting that a test be conducted. Beware however, that a person being called in for testing has the right to know the source of information that led to requiring a test. If you are trying to look out for your parent's best interest and are doing this behind his back, he may find out you were involved and feel betrayed. It is for this reason that you may want to consider being upfront about your concern. Another alternative is that if your parent is pulled over by the police with cause, the officer could site the person for a retest if there is probable cause.

Some organizations suggest that families contact their loved one's medical professional asking them to write an order for a person to stop driving. Although that is clearly an option, be careful. A doctor's order may not be advisable for liability reasons. If a person is given an order to stop driving and they ignored it, or switch doctors as a result, there could be liability issues if the loved one is involved in an accident and it is discovered an order was written and ignored.

State Requirements

The license renewal process varies by state. Only a few states have laws that require retesting at a certain age. Most states only test a person's vision and ask a few basic questions. It is unlikely that a senior citizen would acknowledge any physical or mental limitations that might raise concern.

The Insurance Institute for Highway Safety web site provides information on the renewal process and special provisions by state. For information on the rules and regulations specific to your state visit:

http://www.hwysafety.org/safety_facts/state_laws/older_drivers.htm.
Another elderly driving information source is: http://www.nhtsa.dot.gov.

Additional local and state resources for driving assistance include:

- Local drivers' license bureau
- State Bureau of Motor Vehicles main office *(usually located in State's capital city)*
- State Highway Patrol office
- Local Police Department
- Local Outpatient Drivers Assessment Program *(often associated with Rehabilitation Facilities)*

Questions you might ask are as follows:

- What programs are available to assess if an older person is safe to be on the road. What type of testing is conducted (e.g. behind the wheel, written test)? Is testing required at a certain age or is it voluntary?
- How can a state require that an older person submit to a driving test in order to renew her license?
- What is recommended if you believe your parent's driving is unsafe?

Other Intervention Options

1. Check with your parent's insurance agent for assistance or advice. They might have a suggestion or be able to request a driver's test before renewing your parent's insurance. You might also check with the insurance agent about the liability coverage to ensure the amounts of insurance are sufficient.

2. Talk to your parent and express your concern. Offer alternatives, and help him by providing solutions to see if he will voluntarily stop driving if suitable transportation options can be arranged.

3. As a last ditch effort, I have heard of people intentionally disabling someone's car by removing the cables to the battery, flattening a tire, hiding the keys, etc. These are often alternatives suggested for a parent with dementia, as he may not remember having been told not to drive or realize that he no longer has a valid driver's license or insurance. *Although I am not advocating doing things behind your parent's back*, I am

simply offering these so you have a complete understanding of alternatives. Remember that many of these actions are only temporary solutions and will still require you to face the issue in the future.

> *If you have concern over a loved one's driving, documenting efforts and correspondence regarding your parent's driving may be beneficial. The Cincinnati Enquirer recently reported a story about a man in his 80's who was traveling with his wife, also in her 80's. He crossed the double yellow line and caused a head-on collision killing both of them and critically injuring the on-coming driver. While many states do have maximum amounts of liability that can be collected in a lawsuit for vehicular negligence or a wrongful death, I would hate to have someone lose everything (assets) because of something like this. Even if unsuccessful, being able to demonstrate your efforts to intervene could help you and your conscience.*

If your parent voluntarily or involuntarily surrenders his driver's license, the next logical question is, *"Does he still have a car?"* If the answer is 'Yes,' you might occasionally check the mileage to find out if he might be driving. Even when a person doesn't drive, having a car in a garage may provide peace of mind. When my Mother stopped driving, I asked her companion caregiver to drive the car when she would take mom out for lunch, shopping or when going to the beauty parlor. This was one way I could reduce changes in mom's life and help her feel comfortable by being in familiar environment.

Losing the ability to drive is a traumatic reality that many people will face as a result of age, illness, injury or other medical condition. In cases where driving is not viable and someone needs to change his or her method of transportation, a variety of options are available.

Transportation Considerations

The operating cost of owning and maintaining a vehicle is expensive, yet people rarely give it consideration. As a result, people rarely consider other transportation options that might be available at an equal or lesser cost. The following charts suggest some transportation options and considerations:

Transportation Concerns

Transportation Options	Cost	Convenience
Ambulance *(Non-Emergency)*	Very High	Low
Companion Caregiver	Moderate	High
Family /Friend	Low	Moderate
Limousine	High	Moderate
Personal Car	High	High
Public Transportation	Low	Low
Senior Center Shuttle	Low	Low
Taxi	Moderate	Moderate

Transportation Options	Availability / Response Time	Personalization / Familiarity
Ambulance *(Non-Emergency)*	Moderate	Moderate
Companion Caregiver	High	High
Family /Friend	Moderate	High
Limousine	Low	Moderate
Personal Car	High	High
Public Transportation	Low	Low
Senior Center Shuttle	Low	Moderate
Taxi	Moderate	Low

In an Emergency situation, contact emergency personnel by dialing 911 or the emergency numbers in your area.

Besides the considerations listed in the table above, I encourage families to rank and give consideration to the following more subjective issues.

Subjective Issues to Consider

Other Considerations	High	Medium	Low
Reliability			
Parking			
Flexibility			
Waiting time			
Comfort			
Reliance / burden on others			
Assistance before / after trip			
Companionship while away			
Trustworthiness			
Safety / Security			
Conspicuous / privacy / showy			
Peace of Mind			
Method of payment / Handling cash			
Financial predictability			
Cleanliness			
Special Needs			
Personal and Financial Liability / Risk			

Handicap Parking

When people are able to drive, but find getting to and from one's vehicle to be a challenge, obtaining a handicap parking placard may be an option. To qualify, a medical doctor or chiropractor completes and signs off on paperwork specific to each state indicating that a physical or medical condition merits a handicap parking plaque. In many states, a medical professional also needs to provide a prescription or a letter of request. The prescription usually includes the date, name of the person with the disability, physician's signature, purpose and expected duration of the disabling condition.

Temporary placards are red in color and Permanent placards are blue in color. While both have an expiration date, temporary placards cannot be renewed. A person with a blue placard can renew the privilege by completing and filing a standard renewal form.

Once the applicant and doctor complete the paperwork, your parent then files with the State Bureau of Motor Vehicles to receive the Handicap Parking placard. For the specifics in your state, contact your local drivers' license bureau or your medical professional.

Summary

When personal conditions cause a loved one to reconsider his or her current method of transportation, find comfort knowing many options are available. Although driving is a major source of independence, driving simply may not be a workable option for some people as a result of aging, illness or injury.

For people that do not wish to stop driving, alternatives might be available to help her reduce the amount of driving. For example, if your mother drives to and from a Saturday bridge club, maybe another player can pick her up on the way. Or, maybe family and friends can offer to drive a loved one to and from appointments. You may also be able to provide assistance with grocery shopping and other activities that might create less of a need for a person to get behind the wheel.

At such time you feel it important to address driving issues, realize that you may face major opposition. Don't hesitate to contact local authorities to find out resources and programs that might be available in your area. Give consideration to liability, and make sure insurance coverage is sufficient if a loved one is driving. Consider ways to help a loved one get to and from where they want or need to go, and take time to discuss alternative methods of transportations and determine what might be most suitable and desirable.

KEY LEARNINGS – *Top three learnings from this chapter:*
1.
2.
3.

ACTION ITEMS - *Things you want to do, or do differently:*		
Check when Completed	*Action Item*	*Target Completion Date*

5

Living Environments

People tend to be opinionated when it comes to living environments. Some people say that the only way they are going to leave their home is in a box (implying a casket when they die.) Others immediately think that once someone reaches a certain age, the only option is moving to a retirement community or nursing home. Still others are set on moving in with the children.

This section addresses the many type of living environments and costs. I find that many people are quick to think of the traditional 'nursing home' option, as often they are unaware, or have not been exposed to the many alternative arrangements that may be available. To help you and your family understand the options, and be in a position to make better informed decision, the various environments are reviewed and perspectives are offered to help you determine what may be best for your situation. Emotional implications are also covered, since aging parents can often be apprehensive about change.

Regardless of the situation you are facing, you might find these long-term care statistics startling:

- The federal government's National Nursing Home Survey suggests the average person lives in a nursing home for about 2.5 years at a cost of $144,250.

- The average cost of a nursing home exceeds $50,000 a year. (Source: Health Insurance Association of America - www.hiaa.org)

- By 2030, an estimated 5 million Americans will require nursing home care, at a projected cost of 700 billion dollars. (Source: Mayo Clinic) That averages out to $140,000 a year per person.

As you start considering living and care options, I recommend that one of your first contacts be with the Administration on Aging at 800-677-1116 or on-line at www.eldercare.gov. Visitors to the website enter their state and zip code. Usually three listings are provided:

1. State Unit on Aging
2. Area Agency on Aging
3. Information and Referral Organization

Of the three, I suggest that your first call be to the Information and Referral resource to request information on services, programs and resources available in your community.

Living Environments vs. Care Options

As a result of aging, illness, or injury, many people require a change in living environment or some level of care, either for the short-term or long-term. Often the choice of living environment and type of care needed to address a person's needs or limitations is left up to the care recipient and family caregivers. When assessing living and care arrangement options, it is important to give consideration to current and likely future needs. Also, make sure you understand the distinction between living environments and care options. Living environments are the focus of this chapter. The next chapter is dedicated to care options.

- **Living Environments** refer to where a person physically lives or calls home. For some living environments, care may be provided as part of the arrangement *(e.g. Assisted Living or Nursing Care Center)*.

- **Care Options** refer to the ways a person's day-to-day needs can be met. Care services can be engaged to address a person's unique needs, and provided in a variety of living environments... *in a private residence, in the hospital, rehabilitation center, nursing home, retirement community, etc.*

There are many wonderful arrangements, each addressing different needs at different costs. Evaluating the alternatives and selecting an arrangement, whether temporary or permanent, is a major life decision that merits considerable time and effort. Review and assess the various living environments and care options, to identify the arrangement(s) that best matches your family situation. For families that are not ready to consider a major commitment, like selling a home and moving, care options may provide an appropriate alternative.

Living Environments

A quick summary of living environments follows. After the brief descriptions of each, I provide a more in-depth review of the most common environments.

PRIVATE RESIDENCE: A private residence is often the preferred choice, as *"there's no place like home."* This arrangement is referred to as *"**Aging-in-Place**,"* meaning growing old in the home where a person has lived for years. For many people, this might appear to be the only choice, as the thought of change can be overwhelming. In situations where the physical layout and the functionality of a person's home does not meet his needs, remodeling may be an option. If remodeling, consider potential safety concerns *(e.g. adding grab bars by the toilet and bath, adding handrails and ramps, changing doorknobs and faucets to lever handles, etc.)*

Naturally Occurring Retirement Community **(NORC)** refers to neighborhoods that were not originally planned for seniors, but where most of its residents have remained and grown old. Because of the concentration of older adults, community services might be more readily available.

LIVING WITH RELATIVES: For many families, regardless of personalities, family dynamics, lifestyles or needs, there is no option. Your parents raised you, and now it's your opportunity to provide for them as they age or face an illness. In situations where loved ones move in with a son, daughter, or other relative, a room with or without a private bath is often designated for parents, with common areas being shared.

Elder Cottage Housing Opportunities **(ECHO)** refers to a modular or manufactured home that can either be attached to an existing home, or placed in a rear or side yard. For families limited by the available space in their current residence, or where added privacy is preferred, the ECHO alternative may allow an older or ill loved one to receive support from a family caregiver, while maintaining independence in their own living quarters. ECHO is temporary housing arranged on a monthly rental basis. Make sure to check into zoning and permit issues if considering this alternative.

SENIOR/RETIREMENT COMMUNITY: The terms Senior Community or Retirement Community refer to living environments dedicated to meeting the needs of older adults. Communities that offer the full range of living arrangements are said to offer a *'Continuum of Care.'* In other words, as a person's condition or illness progresses, requiring increased care, a person can be moved from one level or living environment to another within a community, thereby providing uninterrupted care *(assuming space is available)*.

Independent Living – a living environment designed for older adults where a person or couple has a private residence (e.g., single family home, patio home, cottage, condominium, apartment, etc.) within a building or on a campus setting. Living environments may include wider doors, emergency call system, and feature assistive devices such as grab bars in the bathrooms. Monthly fees cover the living quarters, on-site security, and maintenance services. Added services such as house-keeping, meals, transportation, and activities are often available – charges may apply. Costs range from $500 to $5,000 a month or more depending on the amenities offered.

Assisted Living – a living arrangement, often a studio, one-bedroom or two bedroom apartments with a compact kitchen area where general support services are available to address common challenges facing older adults. Residents are encouraged to participate in activities and use common areas. Services include meals, help with dispensing medications, personal care assistance, laundry, activities and other concierge type services – charges may apply. The staff providing assistance is a resource shared by the residents. Access to health care may be available on a limited basis. Restrictions often apply in terms of decorating. Costs range from $2,000-6,000 a month or more.

Skilled Nursing Facility – a semi-private (shared), furnished living environment. Meals and activities are provided in addition to around the clock care Medical care provided by an RN or LPN. Non-medical care is provided by a nurse's aide or certified nursing assistant (CNA). Staffing reflects a ratio based on the number of residents *(e.g. 10 to 1)*. Nursing units are equipped to handle residents' medical, mobility and care needs, on a short-term and long-term basis. Larger facilities often have tiered nursing care units to cater to people that require less care compared to those that require constant monitoring or attention. Costs range from $125-$250 a day or more for basic services. Medicare provides only short-term coverage, and must follow a stay in the hospital.

Specialized / Institutional Care – a living environment (e.g. Hospital, Skilled Nursing Facility Dementia Unit, Rehabilitation Center, Hospice

Center) designated to address the needs of people with significant mental or physical limitations. Costs vary based on the specific arrangement, and can be dramatically higher than a Skilled Nursing Facility.

***Continuing Care Retirement Communities* (CCRC's)** or Life Care Communities. For this arrangement, a person buys in to a community, and is contractually guaranteed lifetime living and care arrangements. CCRC's offer a full continuum of care, and are responsible for providing suitable housing and care based on a person's needs. Communities charge a one-time initiation or entrance fee (usually $25,000 to $100,000) in addition to monthly fees specific to the type of services needed.

> *There is no single best answer or recommended solution. Different families with similar situations often choose different options. When deciding what is best for your family, consider factors that are most important to you.*

How Does One Decide?

Start by making sure you have an understanding of your loved one's capabilities and limitations, answer the three purpose consideration questions below, and then evaluate the various options firsthand.

1. How are the current arrangements causing you to consider other options? What is unsatisfactory?

2. What are you trying to accomplish by making an adjustment to the current living environment or care option? Distinguish between needs and wants, and focus on the needs of the care recipient. All too often families make decisions based on personal wants (e.g. *"I want Mom to live close to my house so I can visit more often."*) Prioritize needs and wants to help you identify the most appropriate arrangements.

3. What are the requirements of a new arrangement? In other words, what is deemed to be essential for a new arrangement to work and meet expectations? If you are not sure, give consideration to the specific issues / attributes you will be evaluating, to know whether the change in arrangements meets your expectations.

Although the considerations and ultimate answers will be different based on each family's situation, the process to determine which alternative(s) might be best remains the same. When answering the questions above, consider your perspective and your parent's perspective. Things that may seem obvious to you may not be as obvious to your aging loved one.

When considering a change, I recommend that all family members involved make a list of what is important to them. Some great things begin to happen when you have a list:

1. It forces everyone to determine what is really important. It also eliminates some of the subjectivity.

2. Families tend to agree on what they are trying to accomplish and therefore, know when they have met a milestone.

3. You will find out what is realistic and what is not as you begin to evaluate the options.

4. You can use the same criteria for current and potential living environments. That may help a parent realize the current arrangement may not be best.

5. You can narrow down the alternatives through a process of elimination to select the best alternative.

Other Considerations

- Does your loved one have sufficient financial means to cover his or her living expenses? I always encourage people to consider their financial resources when considering options. Why? Because one of the easiest things to do is to eliminate alternatives because of financial constraints. By narrowing considerations, it often times makes the decision process easier. (See Chapter #9 entitled Estate Matters)

- Are there medical requirements that require supervision or support (e.g., sight, hearing, nourishment, medication, mobility)? If your parent has limitations, acknowledge them and work to ensure the alternatives that you consider meet her needs. This is a great way to narrow down the possible options.

- Does your loved one have habits that may present a challenge? Common concerns include smoking, volume of television, sleep schedule, overall neediness, and abrasive personality. Communities usually have a screening process to ensure a good fit of the prospective resident and the larger population.

- Are you, your spouse, and other family members ready, willing and able to support a decision? If not, why? By assessing the situation, you will be in a better position to make a decision and clarify the issues you are facing. Decision making is easier when everyone is in agreement and shares a common goal. If everyone involved is not in agreement, be prepared for resentment and the "*I told you so*" type comments. If everyone is not in agreement, go back to the Decision Spectrum and Exercise #2 (both in Chapter #2) to help you find common ground that you can use as a starting point.

One thing my dad always said whenever we began to consider and evaluate alternatives was that "retirement communities are for old people". And, since he did not see himself as old (at age 75); he simply was not going to consider anything except his current living arrangement.

PRIVATE RESIDENCE - *To Move or Not to Move?*

Studies suggest that approximately 80 percent of older adults want to remain independent in the home where they currently live. In fact, there is even a an acronym – NORC – to reflect neighborhoods that, while not intended to be a senior community, have become one as most of its residents have grown old and stayed there. With the popularity of people 'Aging-in-Place,' many communities are developing programs to meet the needs of older adults. As you contact state and local organizations, ask about aging-in-place programs.

Other private residence options include:

1. Moving to a smaller or more appropriate private residence in the same community.

2. Retiring and moving to where ever one's children or other relatives live.

3. Moving to another state such as Arizona, Florida or Maine.

For the adventurous folks that want to move somewhere different and, in a sense, begin a new life, typical decision factors include: taxes, health care, climate, transportation, and cultural opportunities. A couple of websites that provides comparative quality of life and cost of living data are www.BestPlaces.net and www.RetirementLiving.com.

Few would disagree that *"there's no place like home."* Often I hear of people who are noticeably aging and struggling in their current environment, yet they refuse to even consider making a change. For many people, the thought of moving from a private residence where they have lived for years, to a small home or a 500 square foot apartment or room is simply not an option.

If your parents are adamant about staying in their house, as many older Americans are, take the time to access the safety. There are several Home Safety Checklists that can help you know what to consider and assess. One of the most comprehensive is available from the Consumer Product Safety Commission. To request a free copy of the <u>Home Safety Checklist for Older Consumers</u>, send a postcard to: Checklist for Older Consumers, CPSC, Washington, D.C. 20207 or visit: www.cpsc.gov/cpscpub/pubs/556.html.

Retrofit or Remodel

Once you have assessed the safety, you might decide to retrofit the current house so that your loved ones are better able to cope. Consideration may include the following:

- If all bedrooms are on a second floor, can a room on the first floor be modified into a bedroom?

- Consider adding grab bars (similar to those seen in handicap-equipped restroom facilities) by the toilet, bath and shower.

- Consider a hand-held showerhead in the bathroom, and non-slip strip on surfaces that when wet could be slippery.

- In the kitchen, consider a side-by-side refrigerator freezer so height will not be a factor.

- For the range/stove, consider a unit that has controls on the front as opposed to the back where someone has to reach over hot burners.

- For the kitchen cabinetry, consider roll-out shelving in low cabinets.

- In terms of lighting, make sure it is adequate and controls are within reach.

- At a main entry door, add a handrail (and ramp as appropriate) to make the steps easier.

These are just a few ideas for your consideration. I also suggest looking around your parent's home for potential hazards that could lead to a fall, fire or other hazard.

While aging-in-place may be an option for some, it may not be an option or choice for others. Valid reasons often exist that would suggest a need for making a change from the current living environment. Reasons often include:

- Downsize to a more economical and appropriate size home (avoid heating and cooling unused or vacant rooms).

- Find a more appropriate floor plan (possibly without stairs).

- Eliminate responsibility for maintenance (inside and outside).

- Find a home in better proximity to family, friends, social outlets and places your parent frequents.

- Find a home offering more appropriate surroundings (people of like-age).

- Seek a home where support services, activities and social opportunities are convenient and accessible.

- Eliminate unnecessary belongings and reduce clutter while able, so not to burden a surviving spouse or family members with a daunting task.

Some of the major challenges older adults face include inactivity and loneliness. Loved ones may see their friends becoming less active and even dying. Parents usually do not want to be a burden to their children. They often feel it is in their best interest to simply restrict their own activities. There may be better solutions, but they often require making a change. Reasons for making a change to a retirement living setting include:

- The ability to feel safe.

- To have access to resources for assistance as needed.

- To relinquish certain responsibilities such as maintenance.

- To improve the quality of life through contact with other older adults and participation in activities and social events.

- Typical reasons older people do not make a change include:

- The perceived expense of making a change.

- The cost of the new environment *(especially if the mortgage is paid off)*

- Inability to cope with change.

- Concern about meeting new people and making new friends.

- Concern over an unfamiliar environment and new routine.

- The size, type or location of the new home.

If you have concerns over the current arrangement, or simply do not believe it is in your parents best interest to maintain their current residence, chances are you are going to have to convince them that a change is in her best interest. To do that, I recommend you consider the following questions:

1. **What is the cost of your current living arrangement?** It may help to think about it in three categories: Housing, Food & Beverage, and Maintenance. Finances are often an area of major concern for older adults. Also, there is often a difference between the real and perceived cost of living. So, rather than deal with perceptions, deal with the facts. What are the true costs?

EXERCISE #3 – Current Living Expenses	
Description of Expenses	Monthly Expense (Avg.)
HOUSING	
Mortgage or Rent (including taxes)	
Insurance	
Utilities – Gas / Electric / Oil / Coal	
Utilities – Telephone / Cable TV	
Utilities – Water / Sewer / Trash	
Dues – Home Owners Association	
FOOD & BEVERAGE	
Groceries & Miscellaneous	
Dining Out	
MAINTENANCE	
Lawn Care & Gardening	
Pest Control	
Plumbing	
Electrician	
Handyman / General	
TOTAL	

2. **Who would you call in an emergency?** Is there a support system of friends and family nearby? Are people ready, willing and able to drop everything to help? How much time can someone help in a given week? When your loved one mentions someone she would call, write down the person's name and number, and call them to validate that they are

ready, willing and able to provide assistance as needed and at the drop of a hat.

EXERCISE #4 - List of Support Resources
CONTACT #1
Name:
Relationship: (e.g. Friend, Neighbor)
Availability: (Days, Times, etc.)
Contact #'s:
CONTACT #2
Name:
Relationship:
Availability:
Contact #'s:

3. **What is it about the current living arrangement that your parent likes so much?** Talk about it. Try to discover what your parent likes or wants. Often times, what he likes or wants can be accomplished other ways. There is often a fear of change that a loved one may not want to admit it. Only by finding out what he really wants or does not want, can you begin to suggest alternatives.

EXERCISE #5 - Living Environments
LIKES
DISLIKES

4. **Is he able to drive and is public transportation a realistic option?** If transportation is an issue, what happens if your parent needs food or medicine? How would he get to a doctor's appointment? These are real issues. Sometimes people will forego real needs to maintain their independence and not impose on others. Also, give consideration to

who else might have similar transportation requirements and investigate if car pooling or "catching a ride" with someone else might be a possibility. (See Chapter #4 – Transportation)

Another consideration for older adults is the potential for one spouse to be left alone in a home without his or her life partner because of hospitalization or death. Surviving spouse issues are real, especially for women. By the time people celebrate their 85th birthday, women outnumber men by 2 to 1. Women outlive men by five to eight years. (Source: Staci Sturrock of the Cox News Service. Women live longer, not always better. The Cincinnati Enquirer, January 31, 2002) A different article reports that according to the 2000 census, there are roughly 2 million widowers (Men) age 65 and older. The challenge with the men is that they often have a harder time coping with a spouse's death, as they are less likely to confide in anyone about their grief as they fear showing signs of weakness. (Source: Martha Raffaele of The Associated Press. Census shows more older men outliving wives. The Cincinnati Enquirer, December 14, 2001)

The "WHAT IF" Risks: While change can be hard for everyone, a huge concern for older married couples should be: *"Can my spouse manage the household if I suddenly become incapacitated, need hospitalization or die?"*

- Is it a fair burden to leave a spouse living alone in the home?

- Is it reasonable to think that being in a home alone is the best alternative? Will your newly-single parent be able to cope? *(I know that my father managed the bills, handled the maintenance and upkeep issues. When he passed away, my mom was in no position to handle these matters and she would not have had the foggiest idea of where to start or what to do.)*

- Is it reasonable for one spouse to have the burden of going through years and years of accumulated treasures and trash at such time she chooses or needs to move?

The point is, would you want to be left behind? Do you think that either of your parents has the ability to cope if one is left alone in the house?

If you think your parent's current living arrangement is not suitable, you might, besides pointing out the challenges, stress the ease and convenience of moving into a condo, patio home, or independent retirement housing. Comfort them by letting them know you will help them with the transition. Reinforce the decision to make a move whenever possible. Point out benefits such as being around other people of similar age, interests and activities.

LIVING WITH RELATIVES - *All In The Family*

For many families, there is no option. Your parents raised you, and you feel as though you have a responsibility to care for them when they get old. Many people take that stance and that is fine. But it is just as fine to take a stance that says you have a life, a family, and this option may not be in the best interest of everyone involved.

Some things to consider when thinking about this option include:

- Does your parent(s) want to move in with you and your family?

- How does your family feel about the move?

- Can your marriage and relationship with your own children withstand the pressures of someone else being in your house around the clock?

- Realistically, is it going to work?

- Is there space available for your parent? Will she have her own room? Where will she bathe?

- What if stairs become a problem? Is your home equipped to meet your parent's needs?

- Will someone be at home to care for the person? What if you go out of town on business or vacation?

- Will she have her own car or other means of transportation?

- How will the move affect your job, family and finances?

- What respite care services are available in your community to help you?

Having a parent live with you can be a wonderful experience. Do not think by the questions presented for consideration that I am against this option. What I find is that when it works, it can be wonderful. But when it doesn't work, it can be a tremendous burden and a difficult situation to reverse. Just be honest with yourself and your family and try to determine if this will work with personalities, lifestyles and needs. Also, if siblings are involved, gain agreement on the support you will receive from your siblings.

If you invite your loved one(s) to "Move In," do yourself a favor and establish GROUND RULES. _Caution – do not assume._ Is he going to contribute to the expenses? Will he have assigned chores, be responsible for certain tasks or babysitting? When he leaves the house, do you expect him to tell you where he is going and when he will be back? What about his friends visiting?

I recommend thinking through potential issues. For some families it may help to create a family agreement. Part of the family agreement might include expectations of each other and reasons for ending the "live in" arrangement. Reasons often include an inability to provide the needed level of care, conflict not conducive to your immediate family relationship, etc.

Regardless of your position, consider your motivation before making a decision. For example, is your reason financially based, due to a close-knit relationship, or guilt - the thought that they raised you therefore _"this is the least I can do."_

Be careful not to be selfish. What is desirable for you may not be desirable for everyone else in the family. If a parent moves in with you, give some consideration to how he might maintain his outside friendships, stay active with age-appropriate activities, and maintain his independence. What happens when he needs added attention or care? The point is that you might want to plan ahead and think through some of the challenges that may occur.

RETIREMENT COMMUNITY LIVING

In most cities, you are bound to find a vast array of options. You will find different type of communities catering to different needs, some more basic and less costly, and others more elaborate and more expensive. For the sake of comparison, think of nursing home rates as comparable to moderately-priced hotels.

People that pursue retirement community living arrangements are often seeking Simplification, Security, Support and Socialization. A private residence may no longer be practical due to size or layout. Others are seeking to relinquish responsibilities such as lawn care, maintenance and the like. People may want to know that help is available or they may not want to be alone.

Living Environments

Independent living environments within a retirement community offer a simplified lifestyle, and are designed specifically for senior citizens. There are often options involving floor plans, square footage, detached homes, and units within a larger building. Residents may choose to participate in activities and socialize with neighbors, or keep to themselves. Services such as dining, transportation, a health club, and a beauty parlor are often available on a fee basis to complement one's lifestyle. Independent living environments offer peace of mind to family members and can make it easier on a surviving spouse when one parent dies.

Assisted living environments provide many of the same benefits as independent living environments, besides providing assistance with activities of daily living. Assisted living offers concierge-style services where someone is available to provide assistance for pre-determined needs or on request. The key differences with assisted living arrangements are there is little variation in accommodations, and there are often specific rules (limitations) on hanging personal artwork, painting walls, hanging curtains, etc. Residents are charged a daily rate, rather than monthly rent, as is the case with independent living. Assisted living includes basic services such as dining and laundry.

Think about the following when considering a new living environment:

- Making a change can force someone to come to realization that they are 'getting older' or becoming dependent.
- It's often difficult for someone to accept change. Often looked at as what they are giving up as opposed to what they are gaining.
- Adapting to a 'new' routine can be challenging.
- People may have fears about fitting in, making new friends, etc.

Nursing homes are one of the most highly publicized living arrangement options. The Federal Government has spent considerable time and money to rate and rank nursing homes according to a variety of factors. In 2002, the Department of Health and Human Services posted nursing home data on the Medicare website, comparing individual locations with others in their region based on a variety of quality indicators. To review and compare nursing home statistics, visit the Medicare website at: www.Medicare.gov or call 800-Medicare.

Data on nursing homes are no substitute for visiting a facility in person and talking with staff, residents, and family members. The information on the website can be misleading as the ratings can be difficult for people to understand and interpret. Also, the information may not address certain areas that residents and families care most about such as staffing ratios.

Nursing homes tend to be sterile environments and can be difficult for care recipients and family members to accept as home. I encourage you to get beyond the appearance or smell and evaluate the community and aspects of care. Consider the following when evaluating a skilled nursing care center:

- Is it designed to handle medical needs, physical limitations and physiological needs?
- Are activities appropriately based on the level of care?
- Are services available to accommodate needs (e.g., on-site physician, beauty parlor)?
- Are there sign-in and sign-out requirements for resident and visitors?
- Are there secure or locked living areas for people who have a tendency to wander?
- How many people are there to a room?

If visiting the Medicare website, know that senior communities that accept only private pay are not included. Facilities that are represented are those that are certified for Medicare and Medicaid.

Where To Start

If you think that a retirement community or nursing home might be in your parent's future, stop and check one out the next time you drive by. Or, plan time one day to make a visit and experience the community. When you find one or more facilities that you think might be appropriate for your loved one, ask about the admissions process and waiting lists?

To identify retirement communities and nursing homes, I suggest people refer to their local Yellow Pages telephone directory. If you are out of town, many web sites offer Yellow Pages searches. If you refer to a local senior living guide or go on-line to a search websites listing communities, be careful. Many of the publications and website are biased and only list organizations that pay for an advertisement, placement or have some other type of referral arrangement. As a result, it is unlikely that the communities and services mentioned reflect a comprehensive listing of what is available in your community.

When visiting a community, gather brochures including floor plans, activities list, and other information that is readily available. Take a tour if you are interested. Many facilities offer a free no-obligation lunch so that you have a chance to experience the environment and see other residents first hand. Ask about the costs, availability, and ease of moving in and out. Be aware that the person who usually conducts the tour is often a sales person. As such, they may not be reflective of the type of people that work at a community. I suggest that if you are seriously considering a community, show up 15-30 minutes before your scheduled visit and take the opportunity to observe the staff and residents when it may not be expected. Also, do not hesitate to talk with staff members while on your tour.

Specific Questions and Considerations

If an assisting living or skilled nursing care arrangement appears to be a good solution for your situation, consider assessing the following items as you tour communities:

- What is the staff to resident ratio for the unit you are considering? For example 1 to 8 or 1 to 14. Ask if the ratios are the same during all shifts. Staffing ratios are important, as ratios will give you an idea of the level of attention your loved one might expect.

- What is the average length of employment for their caregivers and what training is offered? How does the turnover compare with other facilities you are considering? I suggest looking at the jobs section of the Sunday paper to see which facilities are seeking help. Ask how they handle staffing if they are short of staff.

- Ask about the activities, therapeutic and spiritual programs, laundry service, transportation, and more. While there are no right or wrong answers, compare the answers with those of other area facilities and determine what you think is most appropriate for your loved one. What opportunities are there for family members to participate along with the resident?

Find out what a typical day is like and observe the unit to verify what you are being told is, in fact, true. At one community, I found that during the times between meals, the TV was used as a babysitter. And, instead of watching age-appropriate movies or things like American Movie Classics, it was the talk shows and other "inappropriate" shows. Also, the TV was always blaring so that those who were harder of hearing could hear.

- Ask about the food or dietary services. Do the arrangements seem reasonable compared to other facilities you are considering? Do residents order off a menu or are the meals set? Can family members join the residents for meals and what is the cost? Under what circumstances can residents get in-room service? What level of assistance is available with meals? Is there a separate room for family celebrations?

- Things to observe and look for on your tour: Do the residents seem happy, comfortable, and relaxed? Does the staff refer to residents by name? How does the place smell? Is it clean? Are staffing schedules visible? Is the staffing level consistent with what you have been told? Are handbooks or policies visible or available? Do the policies and procedures seem reasonable?

- Ask about structural or operational issues that might be of concern such as how fire alarms or tornado alerts are handled. When are the exterior doors locked? Is there a sign-out and sign-in process for residents? What about visitors? What type of security measures is in place? How do they handle parking for residents and visitors? How close is the nearest bus stop?

- Living arrangement considerations: Do they offer private vs. semi private rooms? What size rooms and layouts are offered and available? Are residents more often in their rooms or in the common area? Can residents paint their rooms the color they wish? Can they hang their own curtains? Bring their own furniture? Can residents hang their own pictures or artwork? Is there enough space for family pictures and knick-knacks? Is each room individually regulated for heating and air conditioning? What is suggested for phone service? What about cable/TV?

- Care and continuing care considerations: What levels of care do they offer? (e.g., Independent, Assisted Living, Nursing Care, Specialty Care, etc.) Do they offer continuing care so that if your parent's needs change, either temporarily or permanently, her needs can be met within the current environment without relocating to a new community? What is the process for moving a resident from one level of care to another? What input does the family have?

- Is the unit certified for Medicare and Medicaid? If a unit is certified, certain expenses may be covered for a set period of time or when a person's money runs out.

- How are personal funds handled? Does the community have policies for personal funds, such as how much cash a resident should have on hand? Are there special procedures to help safeguard funds? Do they offer on-site banking? What are reasons a resident might need money? (e.g., general store, field trip.)

- Insurance considerations: Should the resident have Liability or Personal Property Insurance? What type of coverage does the community have?

- Admissions Process and Wait List. When you find that you are interested in a community, how does the admissions process work? Are there specific criteria admissions? Is there a wait list? What number would your parent's name be on a wait list and what is the probable timing? Is a deposit required? When is the deposit refundable and not refundable?

- Facilities Policies: What are the visiting hours? If the hours are set as opposed to being 24 hours a day, what is their explanation why? Are pets allowed in the community? Can residents and visitors smoke?

- What is the fee structure (e.g., $X per day)? Are there one-time applications or admissions fees? What are examples of fees that would not be included and billed separately? How much have fees increased over the past few years?

- What happens to a person's "space" if they require hospitalization? Is the space held for a certain period? Is the rate discounted during the time away? Is there a way to maintain the "space" beyond the set period?

- Who is the primary contact person for family? What is his or her title and availability? Have you met them?

Waiting Lists

If during your search you find that waiting lists are common, you may be able to use them to your advantage. Many people delay making a decision until the need is upon them, only to find out there is *"no room at the inn.*" Rather than settling for a second or third choice, engage your parents earlier in the process and encourage them to visit a few facilities to find out which ones he likes better. If there are no available units, a visit can be totally non-threatening. If you find a community she likes, even though she might not be ready or willing to make a move, put down a deposit and get her name on the list. By the time her name does come up, things may have changed and she might be more willing. Remember that you can always say "No" if a unit becomes available and you are not ready to make a move.

Making Your Decision:

You will quickly find that no two facilities are alike and there will most likely be trade-offs when selecting one community over another. I highly recommend you determine the five or ten most important factors, assign a weight to each factor and then score each community. This enables a more objective approach. People are often surprised to see which community's score ranks the highest. Ideally your needs should be the factors that carry considerable weight. Other factors could include such things as proximity to your home, depth and breadth of care options, etc.

EXERCISE #6 - Community Selection Scoring				
FACTOR	Weighting %'age	Facility #1	Facility #2	Facility #3
1.	____%			
2.	____%			
3.	____%			
TOTAL	100%			

I suggest scoring each factor using a three point scale where 1 is below average to average, 2 is average to above average, and 3 is above average to excellent or best in class.

Although I have provided information and tools above, one question I often receive is, "*what were the considerations you had when we selected a community for your mother?*" The following is provided only as a reference point.. Just because these were issues that we deemed important, it does not suggest that the same issues should or should not be important to you in your situation. In other words, take what you like and leave the rest.

Living Environments

STAFF EXPECATIONS:
- *Resident to staff ratio of 8 to 1 or better with at least two staff working the unit at any one time (except 3rd shift)*
- *RN access for medical purposes with reasonable response time (30-45 minutes max.)*
- *Visible staff involvement and interaction with residents*
- *Staff's reasonable encouragement of residents to participate in activities*
- *Staff's understanding of medical conditions, needs and appropriate activities (Not using TV as a babysitter or over medicating to avoid care issues)*
- *Staff presence NOT behind a desk, counter or other "passive" location.*
- *Staff's acknowledgement of residents by name (includes Administration, Maintenance, etc.)*
- *Reasonable staff turnover rate for primary caregivers (avg. tenure over 18 months)*
- *Back-up plan to address staff absences and holiday coverage*
- *Acceptance of and responsibility for residents*

RESIDENTS APPEARANCE & PARTICIPATION
- *Resident's dignity reasonably addressed through clothing, hair care and hygiene*
- *Residents encouraged to be out of their rooms*
- *Staff going into resident's rooms at least once every two hours during normal working hours (if not in common area)*
- *Residents "getting along" with each other*
- *Dignified environment conducive for residents to LIVE*
- *Non-smoking environment*
- *Residents not waiting at doors to "escape"*

MAINTENANCE & HOUSEKEEPING
- *Common areas appear clean and less visible things are not ignored*
- *Garbage picked up at least once a day from residents rooms and unit*
- *Residents rooms cleaned at least once a week (e.g., vacuumed, toilet cleaned, dusted)*

RESIDENTS ROOMS
- *Appropriate size for personal items and belongings*
- *Ability to hang personal artwork and personalize their setting*
- *Acceptable evacuation plan (especially if not on ground floor)*

OTHER
- *Acceptable dietary plan to acknowledge and address Mom's weight loss*
- *Routine – structure in the day-to-day activities*
- *Activities schedule posted and adhered to (not just posted on wall for families benefit)*
- *Acceptable references from at least three residents family members*
- *Family holiday activities*

Summary

If you think your parent's current living arrangement is not suitable, you might, besides pointing out the challenges, stress the ease and convenience of moving by letting them know you will help them with the transition. Frequently reinforce the benefits of living in what you believe is a more appropriate environment. Make sure to balance the needs and perspectives of everyone involved and follow the Golden Rule.

Don't underestimate the challenges associated with change. Imagine for yourself if you were displaced from a familiar and comfortable setting you call home. Besides making a physical change, many people find it necessary to consolidate their personal belongs and get rid of years of accumulated stuff. Remember the saying, *"One man's trash is another man's treasure."*

KEY LEARNINGS – *Top three learnings from this chapter:*
1.
2.
3.

ACTION ITEMS - *Things you want to do, or do differently:*		
Check when Completed	*Action Item*	*Target Completion Date*

6

Care Options

Regardless of whether a loved one is living in his own home, with relatives, in a retirement community or is a patient at the hospital, separately consider the type of care a loved one needs.

Personalized care is a wonderful option, because a loved one benefits from receiving needed care in the comfort of his or her home. Care services are tailored to meet each care recipient's needs, ranging from a few hours to around the clock care. The cost varies with the time commitment, frequency and skill of the caregiver. Since formal (paid) caregivers provide care on an individual basis, the hourly fee may appear high; however, the duration of caregiving can often be limited to specific hours making it an affordable and desirable option.

Many people are unable to care for themselves. The most common type of care people need involves Activities of Daily Living (ADL's). As discussed in Chapter #2, ADL's relate to personal care and one's ability to independently manage the day-to-day life.

By providing assistance or care for someone, the hope is to avoid someone struggling unnecessarily. Recognizing a person's care needs may be challenging for able bodied Baby Boomers to understand. So many of us take for granted our health and our ability to cope in a variety of circumstances. To give you insight into an older person's world and help you appreciate the types of challenges an older person may face, let's use an example of person with Arthritis. Start by thinking of all the different things you do during the course of the day that involve your hands and fingers. From turning off the alarm clock, opening a tube of toothpaste and brushing our teeth, to getting dressed, buttoning a shirt, lacing shoes, preparing and eating breakfast, and more. That's simply the first 30 – 45 minutes of the day. What about turning a door knob, maneuvering your keys into your car's ignition or door, or handling a writing instrument? All of the activities mentioned require manual dexterity. If Arthritis impacts the joints in your fingers and hands, all of these activities could be challenging. If your loved one has a medical condition, focus on the prognosis. I encourage you to use the same line of thinking to help you understand and appreciate the challenges your loved one may be facing. Doing so should better help you to anticipate, recognize and address one's needs.

Whatever condition you or a loved one is facing, consider the type of activities he engages in daily and how you can make his life easier. For families that are unable to provide the care a loved one needs and deserves on an on-going or an occasional basis, there are a variety of care options. Care services are available on a Private Pay, Medicare and subsidized basis.

Community and State Programs

Many states and cities have specialized programs designed to address the unique need of today's older adults. For example, Ohio has what is referred to as the Passport Program. Passport is a home health care program that provides state subsidized meals, personal care, and services addressing other needs. The program was devised in 2001 to be a humane and economical alternative to nursing homes. Apparently, a state-subsidized nursing home bed runs about $47,000 a year compared to an average cost of roughly $8,800 for each Passport participant.

Many counties across the US have Elderly Services Programs (ESP) supported by tax levies. For example, in Warren County Ohio, services include intake, assessment and case management, home delivered meals, homemaking, personal care, adult day services, respite care, electronic monitoring services, medical transportation, minor home repairs, and independent living assistance. Check with your local Area Agency on Aging to learn about programs that might be available in your community.

Government programs are typically intended for residents age 60 or older that have a need for services as determined by a case manager. Services are provided to low-income elderly at no cost. Others are required to help pay for the cost of care, based on a sliding fee scale that considers income and ongoing medical expenses. For programs such as home-delivered meals, donations are often requested.

Care Services and Programs

The following is a list and brief description of the various types of care options:

- **Companion Care,** also referred to as 'Custodial Care,' is personalized non-medical care similar to what is often supplied by family members. Care services are designed to meet a person's unique needs, and can include general assistance, companionship, help with transportation, errands, and more. There is typically scheduling flexibility and the ability to increase or decrease care as needed. Costs range from $15-$30 per hour or more.

- **Personal Care** is personalized non-medical care, providing hands-on assistance with activities of daily living (ADLs) such as eating, bathing, dressing, toileting, transferring, medication management, etc. Personal care services can be provided on a continuing basis or as needed. Costs range from $15-$30 per hour or more.

- **Skilled Nursing Care** refers to personalized medical care. Care services, provided by an RN or LPN, are designed around a person's specific medical care needs. Services include wound care, infusion therapy (IV's), tube feeding, catheter care and other skilled medical services. Costs range from $25-$75 per hour or more.

- **Adult Day / Senior Center** refers to supervised enrichment programs for older adults, age 55+, that are designed to stimulate and engage people based on interest and activity levels. Many full- day and half-day programs provide meal service and transportation. Fees range from $35- $95 per daily session or more.

- **Respite Care** refers to caregiving services offered on a temporary basis that are designed to provide a primary family caregiver with short-term relief, or a rejuvenating break from the constant demands of caregiving. *(e.g., in-home assistance, short nursing home stays, adult day care).*

- **Hospice Care** refers to palliative or comfort care. Hospice is designed for people whose life expectancy is limited, often due to a terminal illness such as cancer. The focus is on providing comfort and compassion during a person's end of life.

- **Adjunct Services** are other services are available on "*as needed*" and "*as available*" basis to meet specific needs who are shut-in, or otherwise unable to provide for themselves. Adjunct services include Shared Housing, Housekeeping, Meal Services, Transportation, and Bill Paying Services.

Most care services can be provided anywhere a family needs care…in their home, in the hospital, rehabilitation center, nursing home, retirement community, etc. To determine which service or mix of services might be best for your situation, go back to "10 Caregiving Considerations" in Chapter #1 and start with an understanding of your parent's capabilities and limitations. Consider all the care options to identify the services that best complement a loved one's requirements and address the agreed on Needs and Wants.

In the following section, I describe each care option and provide insight to help you determine what type of care you might wish to pursue.

Companion & Personal Care

Two of the more popular In-Home care arrangements are companion care and personal care. Companion and personal care services are often provided by one organization or caregiver. The reason they are often differentiated is that some states require certification for a paid caregiver to physically touch a client.

Companion care is best described as care similar to what is often supplied by family members. Many families, especially in situations where a son or daughter is considered a long distance caregiver, hire a person to provide day-to-day assistance and companionship for a loved one. A companion care arrangement often enables a person to remain independent in his or her home for a longer period of time while providing for many of their basic needs. This is also a popular care option among dual income families or in situations where a relative is unable to allocate set blocks of time to help a loved one. For persons living alone or experiencing memory impairments, companion care is often appropriate.

Personal care refers to hands-on assistance with daily living activities (ADL's) such as eating, bathing, dressing, toileting, transferring, and medication management. Companion care and personal care services can be provided on a continuing basis or as needed. There is typically scheduling flexibility and the ability to increase or decrease care as needed.

While many organizations offering In-Home care services provide a long list of everything they can do for a person, I distill the services into the following four buckets. When I refer to companion care and personal care, I am referring to non-medical care:

1. COMPANION CARE – In-home companionship services designed to engage and stimulate people through conversation and recreation.

2. DAILY LIVING CARE – A wide variety of services to help people with activities of daily living including: grooming and dressing guidance, reminders for medication, help with personal matters such as scheduling appointments and organizing bills, scheduling or preparing meals, performing light house keeping, doing the laundry, etc.

3. TRANSPORT CARE – Assistance with errands and appointments, whereby a caregiver provides the transportation and accompanies a person or handles matters for them. Whether picking up prescriptions or groceries, clothes or gift shopping, or getting a loved one to and from an appointment, care recipients often appreciate the personal touch.

4. FAMILY CARE – Services to address family concerns and offer peace of mind. From personal emergency response systems (PERS) to periodic reviews with family and respite care, this focuses on the needs of family members.

Skilled Nursing Care

Skilled nursing care refers to personalized care designed around a person's specific medical care needs. Besides medical care services such as wound care, infusion therapy (IV's), catheter care and other skilled medical services, caregivers are also able to handle personal care needs. Skilled nursing care is also referred to as home health care and private duty nursing. The federal government offers quality indicators on the many agencies or organizations providing in-home medical care, similar to how they rate and rank nursing homes. For information on home health care providers' performance, visit: www.Medicare.gov. Only organizations providing medical care are included.

In-Home Care Consideration

Receiving care services in one's home is often desirable as there is minimal disruption to a person's life. No one has to pack-up and move, and families may avoid having to make major decisions like selling a house. With in-home care situations, a caregiver can tailor services provided to meet each client's individual needs, ranging from a few hours to around the clock care.

Care services are available on a direct hire basis and through organizations/agencies. If you chose to hire an individual, a direct hire, know that there are payroll, tax and workers compensation issues. Contact the bureau of employment in your state for the particulars and filing requirements. Also, talk with your insurance agent about potential liability issues should a caregiver become injured on the job.

Organizations or agencies that provide in-home care services, whether medical or non-medical, usually charge a flat hourly rate. An advantage to working with an agency is that they oversee the relationship and work to ensure a care recipient's needs are being met. Also, as care needs increase or decrease, they have flexibility to adjust hours and engage additional caregivers as needed. There are many in-home care providers in most cities.

The following are questions to consider asking an in-home care provider when evaluating their services. This is a general question set so the questions might not apply to every situation. For example, if you are looking for short-term, around-the-clock nursing assistance, you might only care how soon a caregiver can start. For situations, where there will be one-on-one contact for a longer period of time, all the questions may be pertinent. There is no right or wrong answer to a question. As you begin to evaluate options, you may find distinct trade-offs. These questions are suggested based on the collective experience of people who have been in your shoes, to help assist you with your evaluation:

- How does the organization assess an individual's needs?
- Do they provide you with a care plan?
- What type of supervision is in place?
- What requirements do they have such as a minimum number of hours, minimum expectation for the duration of an assignment?
- Are the caregivers' agency employees or sub-contractors?

- What is their policy on background checks and drug screening?

- Are the caregivers bonded?

- What type of liability coverage is in place, what are the limits?

- How is the agency or organization compensated? *(percentage mark-up, flat fee, etc. Feel free to ask what the mark-up or fee is)*

- What is the turnover for personnel? How does their average compare in your city or community?

- What is the average term of a caregiver's employment?

- What is the level of training or medical designation your family should expect?

- How do they match caregivers with the person they will be helping? Does the family have an opportunity to interview potential caregivers or is a caregiver just assigned?

- What are the most common reasons for changing a caregiver?

- Are most of their caregiver placements for temporary assignments or long-term relationships?

- Who from the agency oversees the care relationship? What is the process should discipline be needed or a relationship ended?

- What back-up is available if a caregiver is out sick, on vacation or otherwise unable to perform her duties? Also, what is the process and typical timeframe to secure a substitute caregiver so that caregiving coverage is not interrupted?

- What payment arrangements are available? *(If you go through an agency, the fees should cover taxes, liability coverage, employment taxes, etc. But, if you hire someone direct, you may be responsible for your own liability insurance, filing with the state bureau of employment services, providing tax forms, etc.)*

- What is the ownership of the caregiver company? *(Find out about the financial solvency of the company. Do they appear to be solid as if they will be in business for some time?)*

- How are family members kept up-to-date on their loved one's condition? Do they offer a quarterly care conference, provide updates over the telephone, etc?

- What services are included and what services are not included? (e.g., assistance with dressing, laundry, dispensing medicine, meal preparation, etc.)

- How do they distinguish between a personal and professional relationship? What safe guards are in place to protect a family from a caregiver intervening in personal and financial affairs?

- What insurance coverage do they have and how are you protected? Do they suggest your parent get additional insurance coverage or riders?

If you choose to hire a formal (paid) caregiver, I have a few other words of wisdom I'd like to share:

- Be open and honest about expectations – we all do things differently.

- Keep expectations reasonable – validate that the caregiver understands what is expected and that he or she is willing and able to do what is expected.

- Give prompt and constructive feedback – we all make mistakes, don't let things boil up inside.

- Don't hold back on compliments.

- Keep lines of communication open.

Paying a Family Caregiver

An article in the June 20, 2002 edition of The Wall Street Journal by Sue Shellenbarger entitled <u>Wanted: Caregiver for Elderly Woman; Only Family Members Need Apply</u>, offered an interesting perspective. *"As more families face the need to care for aged parents and grandparents, some are considering a solution that might once have been shocking: paying a family member to provide care. ......It can be a great idea, as long as there are safeguards in place. ...."* Why would you want to consider paying a family member to be a caregiver? Paying a family member can be a cost effective alternative to getting high-quality care. Also, *"fewer people are able financially to quit jobs to provide free care, as many did in the past...."* Realistically people have real expenses, need to pay the mortgage, etc. *"If that's what you need to do for the care of your loved one, then there should be some compensation for it."* If this is an option that might be desirable to your family, establish safeguards and agree on the role, scope of duties and responsibilities, what is to be considered paid work, what expenses are to be covered or reimbursed, and more. The article suggests that *"A written agreement should be drawn up in advance, and include a pay rate based on the market value of caregiver services, the assets available, and the elder's likely life span. ....Budget for weekly respite care and vacation. The agreement should also include a contingent plan in case the caregiver no longer can or will provide care."*

Adaptive and Assistive Aids

People generally want to maintain their independence for as long as possible. Likewise, people want to feel comfortable, safe and self-sufficient in their living environment. So what can one do when, as a result of aging, illness or injury, a person's abilities diminish and they need assistance?

Fortunately, there are a variety of specialty products and assistive devices that address the unique needs of people with physical and psychological limitations. Additionally, many people choose to modify their living environment so their home doesn't impose limitations.

To determine what might be best for your family, start with an assessment of both the person and their environment. Also, make sure to reassess your situation every few months as needs change.

- If a medical diagnosis has been made, give consideration to the prognosis and how it may affect a person over time *(e.g., dexterity, stability, range of motion, ability to maneuver stairs.)*

- In terms of a person's residence, look at the living environment with a critical eye to identify potential problem areas throughout the home. To prioritize home modification efforts, focus on the things that will make a person's everyday life easier and minimize potential dangers.

To familiarize yourself with the many available options, review the **Precautionary, Protective, and Personal** measures that can be taken to make life easier and safer for an aging, ill or injured person.

PRECAUTIONARY: involves adapting and maintaining one's living environment to address needs specific to a stage in life, or physical limitations due to an illness or injury.

Adaptive Measure often involve remodeling or modifying a person's living environment. Common considerations include:

- **Access**: Wheelchair ramp, secure/reinforced handrails, handrails on both sides of staircases, widening of doors, clear unobstructed pathways, motion detector lighting, low pile carpet, low profile thresholds between doors, emergency exit plan, etc. *(If remodeling, consider making modifications to ensure you have a first floor bedroom and full bath, should maneuvering steps become a challenge.)*

- **Bathroom**: Grab bars by toilet and bath, lever faucet handles, seat in shower/bath, liquid soap dispenser, non-skid adhesive textured strips in bath, walk-in shower, hand-held shower head, non-glass shower door, elevated toilet seat, telephone in bathroom, adjusted counter height, GFCI (*ground fault circuit interrupters*) outlet receptacles, etc.

- **Kitchen**: Lever faucet controls, pullout spray, modified cabinets, adjusted counter height, timer controlled appliances, shut off switches, side-by-side refrigerator, front controls on stove, GFCI outlets, etc.

- **General**: Safe use of extension cords (*not overloaded, frayed or under carpet*), slip resistant runners under area rugs, rocker style light switches, easy access to light switches and telephone, adequate lighting by stairs, in hallways, kitchen and bathrooms, sturdy and stable chairs and couches, regulated hot water heater to prevent scalding, etc.

Maintenance Measures refer to keeping the environment operationally efficient, clean and safe. Give consideration to the following:

- **Frequent:** General cleaning, removal of trash, newspapers, etc.

- **Occasional:** Change out furnace filters, replace smoke alarm batteries, perform as needed repairs, etc.

PROTECTIVE: refers to measures taken to ensure one's environment is safe from intrusion and provides a comfortable and safe atmosphere for a person to live. Two specific areas of consideration are:

- **Structural:** Operable locks on windows/doors, security lighting outside the house, etc.

- **Functional:** Easily operable garage door with automatic opener, working smoke /carbon monoxide detectors, access to spare key, ability to view visitors prior to entry, access to emergency numbers, medications properly stored and marked, etc.

PERSONAL: refers to aids and devices (*e.g. hearing aids, wheelchair, specialty clothing, and personal emergency response system*) that provide essential support to meet a person's individualized needs. Give consideration to the following:

- **Sensory Aids:** Dentures, hearing aids, eye glasses, etc.

- **Mobility and Transfer Aids:** Cane, walker, wheelchair, lift chair, medical bed, etc.

- **Adaptive Clothing:** Front/rear closure garments, Velcro™ closure fashions and footwear, etc.

- **Convenience Items:** Special needs telephone, large handle utensils/apparatuses, etc.

- **Personal Care:** Incontinence supplies, personal hygiene items, etc.

- **Peace of Mind:** PERS (personal emergency response system – e.g. *"I've fallen and can't get up"*).

Once you identify the changes deemed to be appropriate for your situation, make sure to clarify who is going to be responsible to make or coordinate the changes. Also, check with your insurance provider to see what costs, if any, may be covered.

Many organizations provide adaptive or assistive aids. Often, organizations specialize in a specific line of products, requiring people to contact several organizations to address their needs. Solutions for Better Aging is an organization that provides a wide variety of supplies. Knowledgeable representatives are available by phone and can help you assess your needs. For more information, contact Solutions for Better Aging at 888-405-4242 or on the web at www.Caregivers.com.

Personal Emergency Response System

Let me take a minute to expand on Personal Emergency Response Systems (PERS). A PERS can help a person remain independent longer, knowing that help is only a button push away. PERS is essentially a peace of mind service best known by the slogan "I've fallen and can't get up." Care recipients and caregivers can benefit from a PERS. Care recipients gain confidence knowing that help is accessible if they find themselves in an unexpected situation where they need assistance (e.g. a fall or medical emergency). Caregivers and family members gain peace of mind knowing loved ones can access help at any time.

A variety of service providers offer different types of services and arrangements all at different costs. PERS systems offer a variety of devices such as a necklace pendant, wristband, base control unit, or two-way voice intercom. PERS systems are often provided by companies providing in-home care services and by alarm companies. Ask about system range, the ability to set-up customized response options, costs and commitment requirements.

Adult Day Center / Senior Center

Senior Centers located in most communities and select retirement communities, offer what is referred to as Adult Day Centers or Adult Day Care services. Adult Day Centers (ADC) are designed for people age 55 and older. ADC's can be a wonderful alternative for people that either live alone or live with family members, but are home alone during the day. ADC's are also for people who should not be left alone during the day because they are confused, suffer memory loss, have a physical handicap or have a medical condition which requires supervision. A personal interview is often conducted to evaluate the functional, emotional and mental status of the individual and determine if the program is appropriate.

Programs usually offer several enrichment opportunities. Centers focus on keeping older adults active and living on their own. These programs offer older adults supervised recreational, educational, and social programs, and are designed to stimulate and engage people, based on interest and activity levels. Many programs provide transportation, meal service and health-related oversight. ADC's offer family caregivers a respite break to tend to their own personal activities.

ADC's provide peace of mind to family caregivers who are away during the day as they have confidence that their loved ones are safe and not alone. While companion care is an alternative to adult day program, a more common alternative for many people is to remain at home alone all day with TV being the primary source of entertainment and stimulation. Full-day and half-day ADC programs may be offered. Available services and modernization of the facility, where programs are offered, can vary. Look into a variety of programs before making a decision.

Other issues you might consider when evaluating an ADC include:

- Is there a requirement that people have an illness/impairment to participate?

- Is the center prepared to deal with wandering, incontinence, sexually inappropriate behavior, speech difficulties and the like?

- What specific programs and services are available? (e.g. transportation, meals)
- What are the costs?

Respite Care

Respite Care refers to caregiving services offered on a temporary basis, that are designed to provide a primary family caregiver with short-term relief, or a rejuvenating break from the constant demands of caregiving. Examples of respite care options include in-home assistance, short nursing home stays, and adult day care

For more information on respite care, and to find out about services that might be available in your community, visit the ARCH National Respite Network website at www.archrespite.org.

Hospice Care

Hospice offers dignified and compassionate end-of-life and palliative (comfort) care as opposed to curative care. Hospice is designed for people, whose life expectancy is projected to be six months or less, and a medical condition is beyond the point to trying to find a cure or prolong life. Hospice is focused on helping individuals maintain or improve their 'Quality of Life.' Hospice is introduced in this section, as it is clearly a care service, but it is expanded on in Chapter #10, entitled End-of-Life Planning. Hospice can be provided in private homes, nursing homes and hospitals, and is covered under Medicare.

Selecting a Care Provider

Ask around to find out what agencies or organizations other people have used, and gauge whether their experience was positive. You might even ask other trusted sources such as your physician, attorney, care professionals, such as social workers and discharge planners, care leaders at your place of worship and the like. In some cases, I find it valuable to call a local retirement community and ask whom they might suggest. Whenever evaluating potential caregiver arrangements, regardless of type, I always suggest talking to at least two or three. By doing this, you will be able to determine the issues that an agency stresses, the level of professionalism, and be in a better position to determine which fits best with your requirements.

Big Picture Considerations

When considering care options, consider how much you as a family member can provide, and what supplemental services might be needed. One bit of advice is do not overextend yourself as a family caregiver. When friends and neighbors ask if or how they can help, don't be afraid to take them up on their offer. Ask them to help by providing an occasional meal, help with transportation, or stop by for a cup of coffee once a week. I suggest you keep of list of people who offer to help and work the list.

Make sure you get the support and encouragement you need to keep going. Caregiver support groups can be wonderful opportunities to share, learn and grow. People that participate in support groups can help you address issues that are near and dear to your heart, and reassure you by knowing you're not alone.

If a loved one remains in his or her own home, adult children tend to worry and wonder if mom or dad is okay. If a formal caregiver (paid) is engaged, it is not uncommon to wonder if the caregiver will use appropriate sternness when needed to ensure your loved one receives the support he needs. There may also be a fear of a loved one saying or doing something that might offend the caregiver, and you may worry about the reaction. Will the caregiver walk out? While families tend to like when there is a friendship, I recommend maintaining some formality. If you select a reputable agency or organization, they should be able to help you address potential worries and fears.

With adult day care, one of the most common emotional challenges is that you are the cause of your parent's participating in the program. You may even get a comment like, *"why do I need to be here when I could be with you?"* Or for those who do not want to participate, a typical comment might be, *"I do not want to go there, why can't you simply respect that?"* People often forget that social and stimulating activities are essential to helping a loved one maintain his mind and body.

Many people think that when they hire a caregiver or engage in a program that they are giving up something. I encourage you to not look at care options as giving up something, but rather gaining something so that a loved one can remain independent longer.

Care Options

Summary

Coming to the realization that a loved one is no longer as independent as he or she once was is tough reality to face. The good news is that there are a variety of care options available to meet your family's needs. From services provided in one's home, to services provided in the community, I encourage you to explore the many options and determine what is best for your situation. Think beyond the care recipient and caregiver relationships, and give consideration to precautionary measures that can be taken in one's living environment, to reduce the care and support that might be needed. Also think about protective measures and personal aids and devices that might be introduced to provide support.

KEY LEARNINGS – *Top three learnings from this chapter:*
1.
2.
3.

ACTION ITEMS - *Things you want to do, or do differently:*		
Check when Completed	*Action Item*	*Target Completion Date*

7

Legal Planning

Why is it, that even though people know something is important to do, there is a tendency to procrastinate? As I said in my opening letter, information is only power when you apply it and act. If you do not have your personal affairs in order, I urge you to do so. In this chapter and the three that follow, I offer practical information to help you understand and organize personal affairs.

It is estimated that over 40% of Americans age 45 and older do not have one of the most basic components of an estate plan – a Will. A far greater percentage has not executed Advance Directives, such as a Living Will or Durable Power of Attorney for Health Care. Many people that have drafted these and other legal documents have not shared what is in their documents, nor explained their wishes with loved ones who could be appointed at time of crisis or death to make decisions on a loved one's behalf.

I suggest you work with a reputable attorney and review your legal documents every couple of years, or sooner, based on life changes such as divorce or remarriage, move to a different state, or change in employment. If you do not already have a legal advisor, you may consider working with an attorney that specializes in Elder Law. Contact your state's Bar Association or visit one of the following websites for assistance finding an attorney in your area:

- www.abanet.org (The American Bar Association)
- www.martindale.com (LexisNexis Martindale-Hubbell® Directory)
- www.naela.com (National Academy of Elder Law Attorneys)
- www.LSC.gov (Legal Services Corp –refers people who can't afford lawyers to legal help in their area.)

Take the time to talk with a legal professional to ensure whatever documents you draft meet the necessary criteria for them to be valid. Three recent news stories that have increased awareness of the importance of having one's affairs in order are:

1. The death of Dale Earnhardt – *the estate went to probate requiring disclosure of personal and business financial matters.*

2. The death of Ted Williams – *the corpse of the baseball legend became the subject of a family dispute.*

3. The Florida battle between the husband and parents of Terri Schiavo. – *the parents and husband are embattled over life support for a woman who has been in a coma for more than 13 years.*

The documents addressed in this chapter are as follows:
- Will
- Trust
- Durable Power of Attorney
- Advance Directives
    o Living Will
    o Durable Health Care Power of Attorney (also known as a Health Proxy)

I also elaborate on Probate, Conservatorship and other legal concerns including Scams and Identity Theft.

As you will quickly realize, there are many decisions to make regarding one's personal affairs. Everything is not cut and dry. There are no quick and simple answers to the questions of how one's property is to be disposed of following death. Distribution of one's assets depends on the type of property and how property is titled. For example,

1. Joint property with right of survivorship (e.g. real estate, home contents, securities, automobiles, etc.)

2. Contractual property – includes Life insurance, annuities, pension benefits, deferred compensation benefits, trust agreements, etc. The contract or the way the holdings are titled governs distribution at death.

3. Property held in individual's sole name – disposed of by Will or state law of intestacy.

Legal Planning

Will

    A Will, also referred to as a 'Last Will and Testament,' is a legal document that indicates how a person would like his or her personal property distributed upon death. The term 'personal property' refers to financial instruments (e.g. cash, checking account, stocks) and physical items of financial and sentimental value (e.g. home, cars, collectibles, household items). (*For people with minor children or grandchildren under their care, a Will would also appoint someone to care for the minor children if necessary.*)

    Anyone who owns personal property should have a Will regardless of the value. While the word estate may be perceived as something only wealthy people have, in the context of estate planning, the term estate refers to the collection of personal property regardless of value.

    The purpose of a Will is to:

- Detail the family members (children, stepchildren, etc.) and causes or organizations for which the deceased would like to provide.

- Specifically mention someone or an organization for which the deceased intentionally wishes to disinherit or ensure they get nothing.

- Indicate the desired disposition of home, auto, investments, financial resources, collectables, heirlooms, and personal items.

- Assign specific assets either by description, flat dollar amount or by percentage.

- Name a person to carry out the wishes stated in the Will.

    A Will can be a simple paragraph or a long drawn out document. If a person dies and does not have a Will, or dies 'Intestate' as the law calls it, a person's assets will be disposed of according to an order of succession prescribed by state law.

    When drafting a Will, name a person or organization (e.g., bank) to execute the Will according to the specified terms. This person or organization, referred to as the executor, handles the administration of an estate upon death. If an executor is not named, the Probate Court will select an executor. There is a statutory order of preference to guide the Court in making its selection.

While the requirements vary from state to state, for a Will to be considered valid, there are a few general requirements. Check with an attorney licensed in your state for the specific requirements.

1. It must be computer generated or typewritten – *only a few states accept handwritten Wills.*

2. It must clearly state whose Will it is For example: *This is the Last Will and Testament of (Insert name) or, "I, (insert name), now a resident of (insert name of county and state), declare this to be my last will, revoking all prior Wills and Codicils made by me.")*

3. It must be dated and signed by the person whose Will it is. For example: *"In Witness Whereof, I have signed this, my last Will on (Insert date)"*

Signature
Spell out Full Legal Name

4. It must have two or three witnesses that observe the person whose Will it is sign it, and then sign the Will as a witness. A witness cannot be named in the Will to inherit anything. For example: *"The foregoing Will of (insert name) was signed and acknowledged by him as his last Will in our presence, who, in his presence and in the presence of each other and at his request, have hereunto signed our names as witnesses."*

Signature #1
Spell out Full Legal Name
Address: _____

Signature #2
Spell out Full Legal Name
   Address: _____

Signature #3
Spell out Full Legal Name
   Address: _____

5. The directives or wishes stated in the Will should be clear and concise in the event that the Will is disputed.

A Will may be changed as often as someone likes. Changes are frequently made by a simple addition of what is referred to as a 'codicil' or amendment. A Will is valid until changed or revoked. If more than one version of a Will are presented after death, the Will with the most recent date is deemed valid, assuming it meets the state requirements. Statements or intentions spelled out in earlier versions are considered null and void.

Besides personal property that is covered in the Will, there may also be property which a husband and wife jointly own such as a house. Joint property often indicates the names of the husband and wife on the ownership document, such as a deed or title. In the case of jointly owned property, there is what is called right of survivorship, meaning that the property will pass automatically to the survivor when one spouse dies.

Other property which is often handled outside of a Will includes assets that indicate a beneficiary such as an IRA or life insurance proceeds. The named beneficiary (whether it be an individual, multiple people or an organization), will receive the funds or proceeds regardless of what is stipulated in the Will. Assets that are held in Trust are distributed according the Trust provisions and are not subject to the terms of a Will. Also, Annuities are distributed according to how they are titled. Make sure everything is up-to-date.

Communicating Your Intentions

I believe that it is equally important to establish a Will, as it is to communicate your intentions to persons who may be named in a Will. While some families may not wish to share the detail and overall value of an estate, I believe that the intentions should be expressed. I have witnessed a number of situations where family feuds could have been avoided if surviving family members knew a loved one's intentions and desires.

In the February 19, 2004 edition of The Cincinnati Enquirer there was an article entitled <u>Memories spark inheritance hassles</u>, written by Mark Coomes of the Louisville Courier-Journal. He indicated that *"the most populous generation in US history is in the process of inheriting the greatest fortune in the annals of humankind – more than $7 trillion by 2040."* However for many people, the inheritance is not about the money as much as it is the memories. The arguments have to do with items of sentimental value such as the wedding rings, photo albums and golf clubs. The article went on to say, *"The fights can be ugly and they split families forever." "Money divides very easily…Grand pianos do not."*

To avoid family fights, draft a comprehensive Will and indicate specifically who gets what possessions. If a loved one is not sure who should get what, ask family members what items have special meaning or value to them. In other words, ask people what specific things that they want. While Wills commonly address how financial assets are to be divided, personal possessions are often overlooked.

Another challenge is when parents leave unequal shares to their children. An article entitled <u>The Latest Twist on Family Feuds: You Left Sis More Money Than Me</u>, written by Jeffrey Zaslow, appeared in the November 7, 2002 edition of The Wall Street Journal. He said that *"You could take the 'easy' route: equal shares for everyone. But perhaps that's not the fairest way to distribute your wealth. Often times one might consider who 'earned' it or 'needs' it more. To avoid giving well-intentioned gifts that cause strife, estate planners recommend honest dialogue without surprises. Often times a gift may create ill-will among family members. Some parents decide to limit inheritances for very successful children, so needier siblings can benefit. Estate planners call that "punishing success" and say it's usually a mistake."*

If for whatever reason you or your loved one is not comfortable talking about the details or intentions of a Will, another option is to video tape your explanation or write your intentions in a letter.

A word of caution is that many Baby Boomers are up to the elbows in debt and are counting on inheritance to bail them out. An article written by Hope Yen of The Associated Press appeared in the November 29, 2002 Island Packet. In the article Yen used the term 'Waiter' to refer to people who are waiting for an inheritance so that they can pay off their debt. Expecting and waiting on inheritance can be risky. What if your loved one lives a long life and requires on-going care? An inheritance could be wiped out paying for care. Also, you don't want to be caught expecting an inheritance and getting nothing or far less than expected. A story in the March 13, 2004 edition of The Cincinnati Enquirer entitled <u>Businessman leaves most of $103M to charity</u>, supports my point. The article spoke about the estate of Burton D. Morgan which was valued at over $103 million. The article said that *"It was divided equally between the Burton D. Morgan Foundation and the Margaret Clark Morgan Foundation after $10,000 bequests to family members."* I can only image that their three children were surprised.

Legal Planning

Another article that reinforces the point about not counting on inheritance appeared in the March 2004 AARP Bulletin entitled <u>Will Your Ship Come In?</u> The author of the article pointed out that the money people stand to inherit can come in handy regardless of the dollar amount. *"Sure, Mom and Dad will join the ranks of the dearly departed some day, but the reality is that that the day will probably come later and any inheritance is likely to be smaller than you might think." "People who are 65 today can reasonably expect to live perhaps another two decades, and many intend to use that time to treat themselves to long-denied luxuries such as travel, new cars and gourmet dining. In addition, living longer means more health and long-term care costs – costs that can quickly gobble up assets."* The safest best for adult children is to save and plan for your own future without expecting an inheritance.

Probate

When a person dies with or without a Will, his or her estate will go through what is referred to as Probate. Probate is a process overseen by a court where a Will is validated and an estate is settled. Because of the complexity of the probate process, an attorney or bank is often involved or named executor. Administration involves the following:

- Preparing and filing of several legal documents.
- Handling the publication of notices.
- Participate in court hearings.
- Completing an inventory of assets.
- Handling the appraisal of the assets.
- Completing final income tax returns and possibly gift and estate tax returns.
- Handling the final transfer of all remaining assets to beneficiaries.

During the Probate process, a person could step forward and contest the Will. For example, Anna Nichole Smith contested her elderly husband's Will as she was not included, and was not "disinherited" or indicated as being intentionally omitted.

This process takes place in the Probate Court of the county where the deceased person resided. Probate property is all property that is not covered by any contract (e.g. IRA, Life Insurance, Trust), providing for succession upon the death of the owner. The probate process can take twelve months or longer to complete. The value of one's assets can be determined at the date of death or a date six months after death. Whichever date produces the most favorable outcome in terms of taxes is selected. Then, nine months after a person's death, estate taxes (if any) are due. The payout to beneficiaries often does not take place until months or even years after a death.

For personal reasons, people may not want to have their assets disclosed and made part of the public record. When a person wishes to avoid the probate process, a person may choose to place his or her assets in Trust.

The following is an example of the information available in the public records when a person dies, a Will is made public and assets go into probate. (Source: Press Democrat News Services, December 6, 2001, www.pressdemocrat.com/motor/news/06motors_c3.html)

> "*EARNHARDT ESTATE*
>
> *Dale Earnhardt willed his estate to his wife, including everything from his NASCAR race teams to the rights to his name and "Intimidator" trademark.*
>
> *Teresa Earnhardt also inherited her husband's numerous business interests, such as his Catawba County Chevrolet dealership, numerous boats and cars, and their $300,000 Iredell County home, according to Earnhardt's will on file in Iredell County Superior Court.*
>
> *Teresa Earnhardt's attorney, Jean Adams, declined comment, saying she wants to protect the family's privacy.*
>
> *Iredell County tax assessor Brent Weisner has reported that Earnhardt's Iredell County holdings total $43.9 million.*
>
> *Forbes magazine named Earnhardt one of the world's 40 highest-paid athletes in 1999, earning $24 million.*
>
> *A partial list of the assets included in the estate includes:*
>
> *1,000 shares of Dale Earnhardt Inc. Earnhardt owned 100 percent of the company, which has three Winston Cup race teams. The value hasn't been determined, according to his estate inventory list in court.*
>
> *$199,618.76 in cash and undeposited checks.*
>
> *A home valued at $298,230.*
>
> *750 shares of Dale Earnhardt Chevrolet Inc., value also listed as undetermined. Earnhardt had 75 percent ownership interest.*"

Legal Planning

Trust

A Trust is a legal entity established to hold ownership of property and investments. When a person (the grantor) establishes a Trust, he typically maintains control over his assets by naming himself trustee. If a person is a self-appointed trustee, or a financial institution is named, the property in Trust must be handled in strict accordance with the wishes of the grantor as expressed in the written Trust document.

Upon death, based on predetermined wishes and according to the terms and conditions indicated in the Trust, distributions are handled and ownership of property and investments is made to people, organizations and philanthropic causes designated in the Trust. Since the designations are pre-determined, the process is much more simple, expeditious and less expensive than Probate. Plus, there is no need to make a disclosure on public record indicating the value or planned distribution of the estate assets held in Trust.

If establishing a Trust, give consideration to how you are going to fund the Trust. For example, instead of a person having a brokerage account with their stocks, bond, mutual funds and the like, they might want to transfer those assets into the Trust fund. People still have the ability to change their investment mix as normal. It is also important to point out that a Trust can provide for the disposition of the property in the trust, during the life and following the death of the grantor.

Specific reasons for a Trust:

- To hide one's identity and value of assets from the general public. Often times assets such as one's home might be placed in Trust to avoid having one's identity listed in public records.

- To avoid much of the probate process, often saving time and money.

- To minimize tax consequences, depending on how a Trust is established.

- To avoid having to formally disclose one's personal affairs and intended beneficiaries in the public record.

- To provide financial support and long-term care for a surviving spouse or dependent child(ren).

- The ability to name alternative beneficiaries or successors should the primary beneficiary(ies) die before, or at the same time the Grantor does.

- To establish the timing for distribution – either at set times based on the physical calendar or once a beneficiary reaches a certain age.

If a person chooses to indicate timing for distribution, it is often either at set intervals based on the physical calendar or when named beneficiaries reach a certain age. For example, a child named as a beneficiary might be able to have the Trust pay for medical and educational expenses at any time; however, the value of the Trust may pay out 33.3% on a beneficiary's 25th, 30th and 35th birthdays. Caveats like meeting certain age requirements can help prevent children from being foolish with money when they are younger.

Specifics often included in a Trust are:
- Upon death, how the deceased would like for his or her assets to be distributed.
- Handling of Trust A and Trust B components.

A couple of other clarifications on Trusts:
- There is a difference between drafting or establishing Trust documents and actually placing one's assets in Trust. Until assets are placed in Trust, or transferred to the Trust account, there essentially is no Trust. That is why I have referred to the Trust above as a funded Trust. A person may also choose to have life insurance proceeds paid to a Trust fund to control the distribution of the funds.

- Having a Trust does not negate the need for a Will. Even with a Trust, a person is likely to have other personal property that is not 'In Trust'. Therefore, a Will designates how property outside of the Trust will be handled.

There are several different types of Trusts including an Irrevocable Trust, Living Trust, By-Pass Trust, Marital Deduction Trust, Family Incentive Trust and a Charitable Remainder Trust. To learn more about the specific types of Trusts, and to determine if a Trust may be right for your family situation, consult a reputable financial planner.

Trusts are usually administered by a financial institution. Besides the cost associated with drawing up or establishing a Trust, there is usually a nominal monthly charge, commonly a percentage, for the financial institution to oversee or administer the Trust. Financial institutions have published rates or designated percentages based on the value of Trust. Often times, these percentages or rates can be negotiated.

Durable Power of Attorney

There are Power of Attorney (POA) documents specific to health care for personal and financial matters. The health care version is referred to as a Durable Power of Attorney for HealthCare and it is discussed later in this chapter. This section focuses on the POA for personal and financial matters. There is what is referred to as a 'Durable Power of Attorney' and a 'Power of Attorney.' A Durable POA as it is valid upon signature, regardless of a person's level of competency. With a POA that is not a Durable POA; for a person to have authority, they need to be appointed "Guardian" by court order once a loved one is found to be incompetent and unable to handle his own personal and financial affairs.

A Power of Attorney document appoints someone to handle a person's (grantor's) personal and business affairs and make legally binding decisions on his behalf should he be unavailable, unable or incapacitated. Note that for a DPOA, authority can be granted conditionally or unconditionally. Unconditionally enables someone to act on the grantors behalf at any time. Conditionally could be to state that the appointed person has no authority unless the grantor becomes incapacitated or other specified criteria is met.

The range of authority provided by a POA document can vary drastically. Generally, a POA provides authority for holding, managing and controlling all real and personal property owned, and hereafter acquired, by or for a person, and to do things deemed necessary and desirable to protect one's interests.

An attorney can help you understand the benefits and consequences of including or omitting certain language. Common elements of a POA include the following: (An Attorney's wording will be more eloquent.)

1. To handle any legal proceedings
2. To collect and pay debt
3. To endorse or sign documents and contracts
4. To spend money for care and welfare
5. To handle the sale or purchase of assets

6. To borrow money and to renew existing loans

7. To have access to safe deposit box(es)

8. To employ or discharge medical, legal, financial and other professional advisors

9. To handle matters of taxation, including signing and filing returns

It is important to clarify that a POA is a document of Inclusion NOT Exclusion. A Power of Attorney lists a multitude of specific things that the designated person CAN DO. If a POA does not specifically grant authority or permission, then the named POA cannot do it. For example, in my father's document, as POA I was not granted authority to gift money on his behalf. As such, when his alma mater had a fund raising effort for a new building, I was not authorized to make a gift on his behalf. If gifting is something that you or your family might want to consider adding a statement giving the person named POA the authority to gift money. Also, indicate any stipulations such as limiting who would or would not be eligible to receive a gift. (See Chapter #9 regarding Annual Exclusions and Gifting)

There are no safeguards built into a POA and state law does not require oversight. A person named as POA could abuse this powerful legal tool giving them control over a person's checkbook and other assets. One safeguard might be to require an annual or semi-annual review with an attorney or financial advisor to ensure assets are being used for the intended purposes. A POA document and the associated privileges can be taken away if there is suspected abuse and mismanagement. A POA can be updated at any time, assuming the person executing his or her POA is of sound mind.

Advance Directives

When it comes to making decisions regarding a loved one's health care preferences and end-of-life issues, do you know and clearly understand your loved one's wishes? The term advance directives, refers to a person's decisions and instructions about potential medical care. The documents are called advance directives, as they are signed in advance to let medical professionals and others know about one's wishes for medical treatment, in the event that the person becomes unable to speak for himself. An advance directive is not just to terminate care, but also to express preferences for the care a person wishes to receive.

Legal Planning

Each state regulates the use of Advance Directives differently. The Advance Directives that are common to most states include the following:

- Living Will
- Health Care Power of Attorney
- DNR – Do Not Resuscitate Order
- Organ and Tissue Donation

Advance Directive documents are available free of charge through your state. Over and above the standardized Living Will and Health Care Power of Attorney forms, discuss the standardized documents with your attorney and determine if it would be appropriate for you to make changes or additions to the basic forms. For additional information on state specific advance directive documents visit: www.partnershipforcaring.org.

Living Will

The situation in Florida involving Terri Schiavo has increased awareness, and spurred many American's to consider executing a Living Will. In this case, the Florida woman is being kept alive artificially as her husband and parents battle each other in court to decide her future. The 40 year old woman has lived 14 years in what doctor's describe as a *"persistent vegetation state."*

Even with the increased awareness, it is estimated that merely 25% of American adults have a Living Will. A Living Will (also referred to as a Living Will Declaration) expresses a person's wishes about her health care and covers such issues as:

- Would your parent want to be resuscitated should her heart stop?
- Would she want to be hooked to a respirator, feeding tube or other life support devices?
- How does your parent feel about the withholding or withdrawing of life sustaining treatment that could prolong the dying process?
- What are her feelings about medical treatments and surgeries?

Unlike a Durable Health Care Power of Attorney, a Living Will does not require that anyone act on a loved one's behalf. Rather, a copy of a Living Will may be requested when an organization begins providing caregiving services, your parent is admitted to the hospital, or other situations where advance awareness of someone's wishes may be important.

A Living Will is effective only when a person is unable to communicate on her own behalf or when a person is deemed permanently unconscious. The document, which cannot be revoked by anyone except the person whose Living Will it is, serves as instructions to medical personnel regarding her desired treatment. A Living Will can be a valuable tool as it eliminates the need for family members to struggle with difficult medical decisions, and determine what heroics, if any, are appropriate. By spelling out to what extent you want life-support to prolong your life, you take away much of the guess work for family members.

When considering what you'd like to include in a Living Will, I suggest you give consideration to the specific type of medical treatments and surgeries you might want or not want. A resource that might help you evaluate your options is the Five Wishes Document available at: www.AgingWithDignity.org.

The next document we address, a Durable Power of Attorney for Health Care (DPAHC), allows a person to choose who they would like to make healthcare decisions on their behalf. I recommend people execute both a Living Will and a DPAHC as opposed to someone relying on one or another.

Durable Power of Attorney for HealthCare

A Durable HealthCare Power of Attorney, also called a 'Durable Medical Power of Attorney' or 'HealthCare Proxy,' is a document in which an individual appoints someone as agent to make all health care decisions, should he become terminally ill, or ether temporarily or permanently unable to make decisions for himself. This document is only effective if the person cannot express his wishes himself. Many states have prescribed forms for a DPOA for healthcare. If the state form does not sufficiently cover a loved one's medical condition you may want to have this document drafted independently. The completed document must be witnessed and/or notarized.

Besides addressing life sustaining treatment that may prolong the dying process, other issues such as cardiac resuscitation and organ donation may be addressed. Resuscitation orders and organ donation may also be addressed in stand alone documents or be indicated on a person's driver's license.

Legal Planning

Conservatorship / Guardianship

Conservatorship, also referred to Guardianship in many states, is a legal process that serves as a last resort, where a judge decides if someone is no longer capable of managing his or her own life. Conservatorship provides a court appointed person (a conservator or guardian) to handle another person's financial and personal affairs and make decisions on his or her behalf when a person has not stipulated an alternative method such as a Power of Attorney. Conservatorship is often necessary for a person with dementia who is incapable of making decisions for him or herself.

Conservatorship is a process that enables an incapacitated person (a conservatee or 'the ward') who may be unwilling to accept assistance or get assistance deemed to be necessary. The establishment of a conservatorship restricts the conservatee's powers over financial and personal care decisions and provides court supervision over one's care.

A relative, friend, private social worker, attorney, financial advisor, or a public official may petition the court for the appointment of a conservator of an individual. Depending on the situation, a conservator or guardian may be a paid or volunteer appointment. The petition must contain facts establishing why the individual cannot manage his financial affairs and/or make decisions concerning his personal care.

Once a petition is filed with the court, a court investigator is appointed to interview the proposed conservatee. The investigator reports to the court an opinion on the justification of appointing a conservator. If the appointment is ruled by the court to be justified, a hearing is held where the conservatee is given an opportunity to speak for himself. Based on the petition, the investigator's report, and evidence from the hearing, the judge decides whether the conservatorship is granted, to whom and what powers and authorities are to be granted to the conservator.

Ombudsman Program

State governments have what is called an Ombudsman program. An Ombudsman Program is designed to reinforce and recognize the rights of older adults. Programs are designed to provide support and assistance with problems and complaints specific to long-term care related concerns. Services are free and many aspects of the programs are handled by volunteer workers.

As an example, in Ohio, the Department of Aging has a Long-Term Care (LTC) Ombudsman program which addresses concerns about the quality of LTC services. The program works with consumers to ensure these services are being provided appropriately and with respect for the consumer's rights. The program is designed to improve the quality of life and quality of care for Ohio residents who are consumers of long-term care and community-based services. The program also offers information, advice and direction on questions concerning Medicare, Medicaid, legal documents, Pensions, and consumer problems. Representatives of the program handle the following issues:

- Provide legal and advisory services.
- Investigate and resolve complaints.
- Promote the enforcement of laws and regulations.
- Advise and recommend policy to state and federal government agencies on long-term care issues.

Scams and Identity Theft

The unfortunate reality is that older adults are often the target of unscrupulous business practices. Each year, as a result of identity theft or scams, people are swindled out of billions of dollars. In an article from the 6/19/03 edition of The Loveland Herald entitled, <u>Protecting Senior Citizens from Scams,</u> Michelle Scheider, a State Representative (36th District in the Ohio House of Representatives) wrote, *"As hard as it is to imagine, the FBI states that senior citizens are targeted at a higher rate than any other age group in fraud schemes. Every day, someone finds a new way to victimize Ohio's vulnerable citizens. Criminals use phones and mailboxes to reach senior citizens. Ohio Consumers lose nearly $2 billion to telemarketing fraud each year; with about 70% of those victims being senior citizens."*

In March of 2004, one of my neighbors was swindled out of $4,100. They were told they had won $500,000 from a clearinghouse, and once they covered the costs of the filing fees and associated costs they would receive their check for a half million dollars. Of course, they never received anything.

The Cincinnati Enquirer ran a story on August 15, 2003 entitled <u>2 indicted in securities scam</u>. The article written by Cliff Peale indicated that elderly investors were defrauded of more than $780,000. *"One man that invested $150,000 said I was told....that this was the absolute safest thing in the* *world, the same as going across the street to the bank and getting a CD, except with a higher return."*

While many people may find these stories hard to believe, I could go on for hours about the abuse of senior citizens. I suggest that the *'if it sounds too good to be true – it probably is'* rule should apply. Also, remind your loved ones not to believe everything they hear.

Older people are vulnerable and often preyed on because they can either be too trusting of people, or they can be fearful of the consequences if they do not take the suggested action. An article in the July 2, 2003 edition of the Wall Street Journal entitled <u>Annuities 101: How to Sell to Senior Citizens</u> indicated that older adults tend to buy on the emotions of fear, anger and greed. In other words, if a salesperson is appealing to those emotions he or she may have a better chance of making a sale.

Common scams to warn your parent about include the following:

- Unscrupulous contractors who come to your loved one's home for repair or renovation
- "Get rich quick" schemes or guaranteed return programs
- Door-to-door offerings *(Once a persons makes a sale, you may have no way to get in touch with the company. Many are transient hustlers.)*
- Sweepstakes
- Magazine subscriptions
- Also, watch out for Faith-based investment schemes – people saying their doing something worthwhile to do God's work. *(It may be another scam where people are simply pocketing the money. If you have questions, ask a leader at your place of worship.)*

So what can you do to protect yourself and your loved ones from identity theft and scams?

- NEVER pay up front.
- ALWAYS check references.
- DON'T PAY for a prize you have "won."
- NEVER GIVE OUT PERSONAL INFORMATION to anyone you do not know or trust, especially someone that makes contact with you whether it be on the telephone or in person.

- BE WARY of anyone calling to verify personal information.

- REVIEW ALL BILLING STATEMENTS to verify accuracy and legitimacy of charges.

- DON'T ASSUME an organization is legitimate.

- BE WARY of high pressure sales tactics.

- REQUEST WRITTEN INFORMATION so you have time to investigate companies and claims.

Also, don't worry about being polite to someone if you feel pressured. Heck, close the door or hang up the phone!

I also find that behaviors often change as a person reaches a certain age. For example, in my father's younger years, he would never acknowledge junk mail. Upon receipt, junk mail would be thrown in the trash without being opened. When my dad turned 70, his behaviors changed. He was opening all the mail and would even spend the time to read and consider long solicitation offers. He even responded to the many sweepstakes offers buying a subscription believing he would improve his chance of winning. While this may sound surprising, it is not uncommon. As people age, many view the mail as a social outlet. Long solicitations letters may be an opportunity for a person to amuse themselves for a period of time.

Beware of Official Looking Mail

Many older people take their mail seriously. I have heard of so many stories where a person's parents began responding to every sweepstakes offer and read every piece of correspondence to determine what is expected of them. If correspondence arrives that looks official or important, older adults may be more likely to respond, often out of fear. Many older adults simply do not know or do not realize that many official looking mailings are simply junk mail in disguise. Some of my favorites include:

- Important information from the *"Office of the President."*

- Envelope copy states *"Important Information: Please return within 10 days."* Then on the inside of this official looking piece it states: *"Special Social Security Bulletin."* So how do we know it is simply a solicitation? First, it seems like they are trying to trick us because on the envelope and reply card no company name is listed. Instead it uses the words Remittance Center and an address. The determining factor is that in fine print in a corner it states: *"Not endorsed by or affiliated with any government agencies..."*

- An official looking mailer indicates information concerning SOCIAL SECURITY. Then in small print it discloses the name of the company sending the correspondence. On the inside it references a number of pieces of legislation including the names of the acts and house bill numbers, and then tells you what you must do. It also indicates that this is *"Vital Information"* and if you do not return the business reply card within 2 weeks, your request may not be processed.

> *While Aging America Resources does not endorse companies or offerings, I do have a general recommendation in this case. Do not do business with companies whose solicitation materials appear deceitful.*

The fact of the matter is that what many companies are doing may not be illegal. While it may immoral, that may be a personal opinion. The bottom line is that companies do what works to achieve the greatest response. So encourage your parent that as a precautionary measure, they should get a second opinion on offers before responding.

Other sales gimmicks may indicate a *"Special Guest"* invitation and suggest that critical information is being presented. In other words, without it, someone will miss out on something big. Events are often held at restaurants, providing a free meal and ensuring a captive audience. For some events, a person may even receive a ticket.

Another offer is for an insurance policy to take care of *"Final Expenses."* Offers may have a headline like *"Supplement your Government Benefit of $255."* These offers often indicate Final Expenses can be as much as $10,000 and if you purchase this plan (a life insurance plan); you can get a flat amount of coverage (e.g., $5,000). Is this type of plan right for you? It depends. Talk with a reputable financial or legal advisor to determine what makes sense for your situation.

Preventing Identity Theft
Identity theft is one of the fastest growing crimes. It has been reported that in 2003, over 10 million people were victims of Identity Theft.

If you think it can't happen to you, think again. Take steps to protect yourself and your loved ones.

To help protect yourself, I suggest obtaining a credit report once a year to check for inaccuracies or fraudulent use. Also, personal documents such as bank statements, credit card statements, insurance papers, and medical papers should be shred. Shred anything with account numbers, a social security number, birth date, and the like.

The February 23, 2005 edition of USA Today, John Waggoner in his story entitled <u>Dodging some ID theft not so easy</u>, suggests that monitoring your credit report is your best defense as identity thieves typically open new accounts, rather than scamming current accounts. He also makes reference to the Fair Credit Reporting Act and reminds us that residents in many states, mostly in the West, can get a free credit report every 12 months. By September 1, 2005, everyone in the US will be entitled to a free credit report once a year.

Taking Action

If you find yourself caught in a scam, or having had your identity stolen, contact your local authorities immediately. Refer questions about scams, fraud and identity theft to your state's Attorney General's Office. If you find it necessary to send any type of complaint correspondence to a company that is bothering you, harassing you, or suggesting you owe them money for something that you never purchased or ordered, I suggest that correspondence be copied to the state's Attorney General's office and your local congressman. Whenever I have done this on behalf of an older adult who was "getting harassed," the issue has been resolved!!

Big Picture Considerations

If your parent has not prepared any or all of the legal documents referenced in this chapter, you might encourage them to get their personal matters in order. It can be a tremendous struggle when you know that it is in your parent's best interest to complete the documents yet, your parent is stubborn or for some reason *(possibly he may not want to incur the cost)*, he does not find these issues merit his attention. I encourage you to tell your parent of the consequences of not expressing his wishes and the burden it places on a spouse, you and your siblings.

Legal Planning

If your loved one's wishes are not clearly documented, the burden may be on you, another family member, or other advisor to make decisions regarding her medical care. Any decision to proceed with or avoid medical care or medical procedures has the potential to impact her functioning level, care needs and living arrangement.

Summary

Know where your loved one's important papers are kept (e.g., Will, Trust document, long-term care insurance policy, life insurance policy, instructions for funeral and burial arrangements, recent tax returns, property deeds, securities, etc.)

Make sure there are multiple signed copies of a Durable Power of Attorney, Living Will and Durable Power of Attorney for Health Care. You may need to provide copies of these documents to Medical Professionals and hospitals. Also, if you file documents on behalf of a loved one, such as a tax return, you may be required to include an original POA with a filing.

Give consideration to where to keep the original copy of a Will. Many people choose to maintain an original copy of their legal documents in a safe deposit box at a bank, with your attorney, or in a filing cabinet at home. If you keep the originals in a safe deposit box, make sure to keep a copy elsewhere as upon death, the safe deposit box is often not accessed until after the funeral. If a funeral has been pre-arranged or pre-paid, make sure that a copy of the plans and a receipt are available and accessible. Also, make sure at least one trusted person knows where everything is located.

As I mention in Chapter #9, make sure beneficiary designations on retirement accounts and life insurance policies are up-to-date and annuities are titled correctly taking succession into account. Also, remember that documents indicating a beneficiary are handled outside of Will and a person's Trust, if one is in place.

Legal matters are applicable to all people over the age of 18. If you do not have your personal affairs in order, there is no time like the present to get started. All too often, people acknowledge that legal documents need to be drafted, however, they decide to do it later and never get around to it.

Encourage your parent to NEVER buy or sign-up for anything on the spot. Whenever I met with someone offering something for my mother, I would often start the conversation with a statement like, "*Just so you know,*

I am not in a position to make a decision today." If they press on it, I may tell them that my sister has to agree or we always review everything with my parent's attorney before making any decisions. If a company or organization offers you a special deal if you commit today, chances are it is not a good deal. Think about how many people have fallen for that same type of gimmick when they walk into a health club and walk out with a long-term contract. Also, advise your parent NEVER to give out personal information to anyone that calls you on the telephone or makes a visit to your home.

KEY LEARNINGS – *Top three learnings from this chapter:*
1.
2.
3.

ACTION ITEMS - *Things you want to do, or do differently:*		
Check when Completed	*Action Item*	*Target Completion Date*

8

Government Programs

There is often a lot of confusion surrounding Government programs for a couple of reasons. First, the programs are complex. Second, the average family caregiver is in her mid-40's and has no personal knowledge, understanding or experience with Social Security, Medicare or other programs. As a result many people do not know what to expect, the level of coverage that is available, and what type of services are either not available or not covered.

In this section, I address the predominant aspects of Social Security, Medicare, Medicaid, Senior HMO Plans, and introduce a number of other government resources that might be of interest. If your loved one has served in the Military, he or she might be eligible for healthcare and other services through the Veterans Administration.

Similar to Open Enrollment periods when employees make their benefit elections, many of the Government programs have periods of time, or windows, that one must apply for services. If you miss the designated enrollment period, you may have to wait until the next enrollment period.

While I make every effort to distill the volumes and volumes of information into a 20 page chapter, refer any questions to the appropriate branch or department of the government. To start, I have provided a listing of federal government resources that address issues impacting America's older adults. You might also want to inquire about state government resources to learn about programs operated at the state level such as Medicaid.

For a web site to have a URL that ends in ".gov" it must be a federal or state government branch, office or program. In addition to the resources listed, also refer to your local telephone directory for local offices and numbers. In many telephone directories there is now a section dedicated to Federal, State, County and City offices.

Branch/Department & Website	Brief Description
Administration on Aging (AOA) www.aoa.dhhs.gov	Provides general information on aging.
Agency for HealthCare Research and Quality www.ahrq.gov	Provides some of the more recent results from surveys and studies.
Centers for Disease Control and Prevention www.cdc.gov	Provides information and services to protect people's health and safety.
Centers for Medicare & Medicaid Services www.cms.hhs.gov	Provides information pertaining to Medicare and Medicaid programs.
Department of Health & Human Services www.os.dhhs.gov	Provides information and links for various topics.
Department of Veterans Affairs www.va.gov	Provides information specific to U.S. Veterans.
ElderCare Locator www.eldercare.gov	Provides listings for state and local Aging Agencies.
Food and Drug Administration Home Page www.fda.gov	Provides information pertaining to products regulated by the FDA.
First Gov www.firstgov.gov	Provides information and links to many government services.
First Gov for Consumers www.consumer.gov	Provides consumer information resources and includes a Health link providing Aging and Elder Care information.
First Gov for Seniors www.seniors.gov	Provides links to government services dedicated to Senior Citizens.

Healthfinder www.healthfinder.gov	Provides a library of 'reliable health information'.
Internal Revenue Service www.irs.gov	Provides information related to matters of taxation.
Medicare www.medicare.gov	Provides information on Medicare.
Medicaid www.cms.hhs.gov/medicaid	Provides information on Medicaid.
National Institute on Aging www.nia.nih.gov	Provides information specific to aging research.
Social Security Administration www.ssa.gov	Provides information on Social Security.
U.S. House of Representatives www.house.gov	Provides information and links for the U.S. House of Representative.
U.S. Senate www.senate.gov	Provides information and links for the U.S. Senate.

Veterans' Benefits

If a member of your family is a Veteran or the surviving spouse of a Veteran, contact the Veterans Administration at 800-827-1000 or on the web at www.VA.gov to inquire about compensation, health, burial and other benefits specific to Veterans.

Social Security

Social Security is complex with many caveats, special circumstances and exceptions. An overview of Social Security is intended to provide you with an understanding the available benefits and coverage, and to help you make educated decisions to support your loved one.

The source of information for much of this section is the Social Security Administration, their various publications and websites. If you'd like more detailed information or have questions specific to your situation, contact the Social Security Department. In addition to their web site and toll-free telephone number, you might also look in your local telephone directory to find a Social Security office near you.

Social Security's Internet Website - www.ssa.gov
Social Security's Toll-Free Number - 1-800-772-1213

If you contact the Social Security Administration on behalf of your parent, be prepared to verify that you have your parent's permission to discuss her personal matters. You might expect that a representative will:

1. Ask to speak to your parent to ensure they have permission to speak with you, or

2. Require you to produce a Power of Attorney or some other written consent indicating your authorization.

Social Security is divided under five major buckets. Due to the complexity of the information, I focus on topics directly related to older adults. The Social Security buckets and a brief description of each are as follows:

Social Security (SS) Buckets	Description
Retirement	SS pays out monthly cash benefits for eligible persons with enough SS credits earned while working. Depending on a number of factors - such as year a person was born – your parent may start collecting the benefit at age 62, 65 or 67. For example, if a person was born before 1938, the effective retirement age is 65. However, for a person born in 1960 or later, the age is 67. There are options to collect a reduced benefit as early as age 62, and added benefits if your parent delays collecting benefit until age 70. *How does one earn credit? As your parent worked and paid taxes throughout his life, he earned credits that are associated with his SS#. Based on the rules at the time, he could earn one credit each calendar quarter for qualified employment. To qualify for the monthly Social Security award payment, he needs to have accumulated 40 credits. Different credit requirements are in place for people to qualify for disability or survivor benefits.*
Survivors	When a person dies, the Government makes a special one-time payment of $255 to help cover funeral

	expenses. Additionally, if he earned enough SS credits while working, family members including a widow and children may be eligible for benefits. Some of the caveats have to do with minor children and the age of the surviving spouse. Other provisions apply if the surviving spouse is disabled, or if there are disabled children being cared for by the parent.
Medicare	Medicare is divided into two parts: Part A and Part B. If your parent is receiving Social Security, he should also qualify for Medicare. Part A is Hospital Insurance that pays toward inpatient hospital care, *qualified* skilled nursing facility care, *qualified* home health care, *qualified* hospice care and blood provided at a hospital or skilled nursing facility during a covered stay. Part A is the same for everyone and has nothing to do with earned credits or amounts people have individually paid into SS. Part B is Medical Insurance that pays toward outpatient hospital visits, doctor visits and various other medical services. Participants pay monthly premiums that are deducted from their Social Security payments. Think of Medicare as being similar to the health insurance people receive from their employer - except that it is divided into two parts. Parts A & B may not cover the total cost or "pay in full." As such, people may choose to purchase supplemental coverage. Refer to the *Medicare & You Handbook* that participants receive, to determine specific coverage.
Disability	Disability coverage is, for the most, part intended for working Americans who are under the age of 65. To qualify a person must have a severe physical or mental impairment that prevents him from earning a living or a condition that is expected to result in death.
Family Benefits	If one parent is eligible for retirement or disability benefits, and the spouse is at least age 62, he may also be eligible to receive benefits. Again, there are many caveats so consult a professional for specifics directly related to your situation.

Initiating Retirement Benefits

The Social Security Administration suggests that people apply 90 days before the date they wish to begin receiving their retirement benefits. Regardless of when your parent elects to start receiving monthly Social Security payments, everyone should sign up to begin receiving Medicare coverage 3 months before her 65th birthday.

When our mother turned 65, we attempted to seek the medical advice and care of a physician specializing in dementia. Much to our surprise, the physician would not see her until she had proof that her Medicare coverage had begun and she could produce her card. My sister and I even agreed to take full responsibility for the billing until the time that she received her Medicare card. The service provider refused our money indicating they are not set up to bill that way. The point of the story is that you should apply prior to your parent's 65th birthday so the coverage is in effect when he or she turns 65.

The following information is required when a person applies for Social Security benefits:

- Social Security number
- Birth certificate
- Most recent year's tax return
- Military discharge papers (if applicable)
- Name of Bank, Account Number and Routing Number (for direct deposit)
- Proof of U.S. citizenship or lawful alien status for people born outside of the U.S.

Do not forget to report changes of address and changes to any bank account that could impact the direct deposit of a Social Security benefit check.

"Supplemental" Retirement Income

Social Security is designed to supplement a person's other income and, for most people, will not provide a sufficient stream of income for which to live. Hopefully your loved one has other income such as a pension plan, individual retirement account, savings, or other assets and investments that make up the difference in living expenses. (See Chapter #9)

Government Programs

As of January 2005 the average Social Security benefits are as follows:

Average, all retired workers	$955/mo or $11,460/year
Average, couple (where both are receiving benefits)	$1,574/mo or $18,888/year

The numbers indicated represent the average. Find out the exact amount your parent can expect and then make sure you deduct the monthly Medicare premium of $78.20 for Medicare coverage.

The annual budget for Social Security benefits is more than $500 Billion. As more and more Baby Boomers reach retirement age and start collecting benefits, the annual budget is expected to increase dramatically.

What is Due My Parent?

For adults not yet receiving Social Security benefits, approximately 90 days before their birthday, your parent should receive a form that indicates "Your Social Security Statement" form SSA-7005. The form lists the name of the person for which the information pertains.

Based on the most current and up-to-date earning records, the second page of the form projects a person's Retirement benefit at ages 62, 67, and 70. Additionally, it projects a person's Disability benefit, Family benefit, Survivors benefit and indicates whether the person has sufficient credits to qualify for Medicare at age 65.

Once a person begins receiving Social Security benefits, form SSA-7005 is no longer sent. If you wish to obtain a copy of this form, contact the Social Security administration and request form SSA-7004.

At such time as your parent begins to receive retirement benefits, the payment date is determined by their birth date.

Date of Birth (e.g., 1/21/31 = 21)	SS benefits paid on
1-10	Second Wednesday
11-20	Third Wednesday
21-31	Fourth Wednesday

If you receive benefits as a spouse, your benefit payment date will be determined by your spouse's birth date. Once the date you receive your benefits is determined, it should not change.

Simply stated, a person's Social Security benefit is based on a percentage of lifetime wages that are directly associated with his Social Security number. While the 'rate of return' is higher for people with a lower income than a higher income, the rule of thumb is that a typical person will receive benefits equal to 40% of his or her average lifetime earnings.

Once a person starts collecting Social Security, during the 4th quarter, the Social Security Administration will send them a letter indicating *"Your New Benefit Amount."* It specifically lists the new monthly amount, the amount that will be deducted for Medicare, and the amount that will be deposited into your parent's bank account.

When to Take Social Security

While people can begin receiving a reduce Social Security benefit as early as age 62, it may be worth holding out longer, if possible, so that the monthly benefit is larger. The risks you should consider include:

1. The rate of inflation
2. Life expectancy
3. Market conditions (Bull or Bear market)
4. Ability to manage your portfolio

The one variable that I encourage you give considerable thought to is life expectancy. If a person is a poor health and may have a shorter life expectancy, taking Social Security early may make sense financially. If you expect to live a long life, delaying benefits may result in a higher monthly reward, paid out over a longer period of time. One way to assess your situation is to work up a break-even calculation to help you understand at what age, the total realized benefit is more or less depending on if a loved one starts taking Social Security at age 62, 65 or later. Another consideration when determining your Social Security start date is the survivor benefits that your spouse may receive. Delaying benefits may result in less of a benefit for you, however, by waiting and receiving a higher benefit, a spouse may be able to collect the spouse's benefit if that amount is higher.

Taxing Benefits: It is a Give and Take

Many of our parents will not receive their Retirement benefits free and clear. Remember that lovely word – TAXES. Encourage your parent to speak with his legal or financial advisor to understand the tax implications specific to his financial situation.

Social Security recipients are not required to have federal taxes withheld, however that is an option for those not wishing to pay quarterly estimated tax payments.

In terms of determining the "earned income" from Social Security, recipients will receive a Social Security Benefit Statement (Form SSA-1099) each January that indicates the benefits received in the previous year. This is essentially a 1099 form just like other forms people receive from financial institutions for tax purposes.

What Happens when One Parent Dies?

Social Security benefits are paid one month in arrears, meaning that a payment made in February is the award for January. There is no Social Security benefit payable for the month a person dies. Whether a loved one dies on the 1st or 30th of the month, if a payment is received the next month, it must be returned.

When a person dies, the spouse or the deceased's estate will receive a one-time payment of $255 to help cover funeral expenses.

If a surviving spouse was receiving a Social Security benefit that was less than the amount of the deceased, he or she may be entitled to the higher amount. For example, let's say your father passes away. Assuming the monthly amount of his Social Security exceeded the amount your mother was receiving; your mother may now be entitled to your father's benefit as a widow. In fact, the Social Security claim number may actually become your father's SS# followed by the letter "D" indicating deceased.

Medicare

Medicare is federal health insurance program for people 65 and older (and for people with disabilities) that is funded in part by our FICA (Federal Insurance Contributions Act) taxes. It provides *basic* protection against the cost of health care. In other words, *it doesn't cover all medical expenses or the cost of most long-term care.*

The Medicare Program is operated by The U.S. Department of Health and Human Services. The agency in charge of the program is referred to as the Centers for Medicare and Medicaid. Contact information is as follows:

Medicare's Internet Website - www.medicare.gov
Medicare's Toll-Free Number - 1-800-633-4227

Each year, the U.S. Department of Health and Human Services sends eligible households a handbook entitled Medicare & You. The 2004 handbook is over 80 pages, so I hope you are ready for some easy reading. *(That was a joke.)* I have distilled the information down and highlight the critical aspects pertinent to most older adults.

As stated above, there are two parts of Medicare: Part A - Hospital Insurance and Part B - Medical Insurance. Anyone who is eligible for free Medicare hospital insurance (Part A) can enroll in Medicare medical insurance (Part B) by paying a monthly premium. In addition to the monthly premiums, people can also expect to pay out-of-pocket costs such as deductibles or co-insurance. The monthly premiums, deductibles and co-insurance for Medicare change year-to-year. For the most up-to-date information, contact the Social Security Administration.

Initiating Benefits
Three months before your parent's 65th birthday is when he becomes eligible for hospital insurance (Part A). At that time, he will have a six-month period (referred to as an "Initial Enrollment Period) to sign up for medical insurance (Part B). When your parent receives his red, white and blue Medicare card, it will list the effective date(s) and indicate whether the person is enrolled for Part A, Part B or both. A Medicare card is similar to a health insurance card you might currently carry. Just as you must show your insurance card prior to any medical treatment, so must your parent show his Medicare card.

If your parent does not enroll during the Initial Enrollment Period, he must wait until the next "General Enrollment Period" which is January 1 through March 31. If a person enrolls during that time, his coverage will not begin until July of that same year. Also, if a person does not enroll during the Initial Enrollment period, his premium may be slightly higher at the time he does enroll.

At the age of 65, if your parent is covered under an Employer Group Health Plan, different rules and enrollment requirements may apply. Check with Medicare for the specifics.

What Medicare Covers
Hospital Insurance (Part A)

Medicare hospital insurance pays toward the following:

Coverage	Description of Benefits
Inpatient hospital care	If your parent requires inpatient care, Part A Hospital Insurance helps pay for up to 90 days in any Medicare-participating hospital during each benefit period. Part A pays towards covered services for the first 60 days, minus any deductibles or co-pays. For days 61 through 90, your parent will be responsible for paying an additional daily co-insurance amount.
	If your parent requires more than 90 days of inpatient care during any benefit period, he will have the option to use what is referred to as "reserve days." The government awards each Medicare recipient with 60 reserve days that he can elect to use anytime during his lifetime.
	In terms of a benefit period, a person must be out of the hospital for at least 60 consecutive days before a new 90-day benefit period starts all over again.
Skilled nursing facility care following a hospital stay	If your parent requires inpatient skilled nursing or rehabilitation services after a hospital stay and meets the various criteria, hospital insurance will help pay for up to 100 days in a Medicare-participating skilled nursing facility for each benefit period.
	Hospital insurance pays towards covered services for the first 20 days. Then for the next 80 days, your parent will be responsible for paying a daily co-insurance amount.

Home health care	If your parent's health problems limit her ability to be away from home and she meets the various criteria, Medicare can pay towards home health visits from a Medicare-participating home health agency. There is no limit to the number of covered visits your parent can have.
	If your parent requires one or more of the services Medicare pays for, then hospital insurance also pays towards part-time or intermittent services of home health aides, occupational and physical therapy, medical social services and medical supplies and equipment.
Hospice care	Medicare hospital insurance pays toward hospice care for terminally ill beneficiaries if the care is provided by a Medicare-certified hospice and your parent meets the various criteria.
	One of the stipulations is that your parent's doctor must certify that your parent is in fact terminally ill and is not expected to live longer than six months.
	As a hospice patient, your parent can get hospice care for two 90-day periods followed by an unlimited number of 60-day periods. At the start of each care period, her doctor must certify that she is terminally ill in order to be qualified for coverage. As long as your parent's doctor re-certifies that she is terminally ill, her hospice care can continue into another care period without interruption.

A benefit period applies for inpatient hospital care, skilled nursing facility care and hospice care. It does not apply to home health care. A benefit period starts the day your parent enters an approved hospital or care facility and ends when he has been out of the hospital or other facility primarily providing skilled care for a consecutive 60-day period. *(As such, it does not cover Long-Term Care needs should that be required)* There is no limit to the number of benefit periods for hospital and skilled nursing facility care.

Medical Insurance (Part B)

Medicare medical insurance pays towards doctors' services and various other medical services and supplies not covered by the hospital insurance part of Medicare. Once your parent has reached the annual medical insurance deductible, Medicare will generally pay 80% of the approved charges for covered services during the rest of the year. Your parent is responsible for paying the remaining 20% of the cost referred to as co-insurance and any charges not covered by Medicare Part B.

Medical Insurance (Part B) covers:	Part B does NOT cover:
• inpatient medical care • outpatient hospital care • inpatient and outpatient medical supplies • ambulance services • X-rays • laboratory tests • durable medical equipment, such as wheelchairs and home orthopedic beds • services of certain highly qualified professionals that are not doctors • physical and occupational therapy • speech therapy • partial hospitalization for psychiatric medical attention • home attention if you do not have part A • blood • screening mammograms * • Pap smears * • pelvic and breast examinations * • diabetes glucose monitoring and education • colorectal cancer screenings * • bone mass measurements * • flu, Hepatitis B and pneumococcal pneumonia shots* • glaucoma testing * * - specific limitations apply for frequency of examination or testing.	• custodial care (*see definition below*) • most nursing home care (long-term care) • dental care and dentures • cosmetic surgery • orthopedic shoes • routine checkups and the tests directly related to these checkups (some screening, Pap smears and mammograms are covered) • most immunization shots (some flu and pneumonia shots are covered) • most outpatient prescription drugs (*See Prescription Drugs heading below*) • routine foot and eye care • tests for, and the cost of, eyeglasses or hearing aids • routine or annual physical exam • acupuncture • personal comfort items, such as a phone or TV in your hospital room • services provided outside the United States

Medicare also helps cover the health related procedures and costs indicated below. For any procedure or treatment, contact Medicare and ask about coverage.

- Artificial eyes and limbs
- Braces – arm, leg, back, and neck
- Chiropractic service (limited)
- Kidney dialysis
- Transplants (under certain conditions)
- X-rays, MRI's, CT scans, EKGs and some other diagnostic testing

Custodial Care is care that can be given safely and reasonably by a person who is not medically skilled, and that is given mainly to help the patient with daily living. Examples include help with walking, bathing and dressing. Even if your parent is in a participating hospital or skilled nursing facility, or they are receiving care from a participating home health agency, Medicare does **not** cover the cost of care if it is mainly custodial.

When your parent enrolls in Medicare Part B, talk with any other insurance companies who might be providing coverage to your parent. There might be a change in policy premiums, a need to determine which policy will pay first versus which will provide supplemental coverage, etc.

Managed Care Plans

Seniors have choices, and Medicare beneficiaries may select a Senior HMO type plan for their healthcare services as opposed to Medicare. This should be a decision your parent makes based on his health needs, experience, and advice of his healthcare advisor(s). All Medicare Managed Care Plans that are under contract with Medicare are required to provide the same minimum level of hospital and medical benefits.

According to a recent article in the New York Times by Robert Pear entitled <u>HMOs to get more funds from Medicare</u>, while private-plan participation has declined in recent years, the federal government wants to triple enrollment in private plans within 3 years. *"From 1999 to 2003, health plans dropped more than 2.4 million Medicare beneficiaries. Some pulled out of Medicare entirely, while others curtailed their participation by withdrawing from specific counties. About 4.6 million beneficiaries, or 11% of the 41 million people enrolled in Medicare, are now in HMOs, which have customarily provided drug benefits and preventive care, not available in the original fee-for-service program. The number of people in private plans reached a peak of 6.3 million, or 16 percent of beneficiaries, in late 1999."* In an effort to encourage private health plan providers to enter the Medicare arena, the federal government is increasing payments to health maintenance organizations by a record 10.6 percent in addition to encouraging providers to increase benefits for the elderly.

Medicare HMO or Senior HMO plans are offered by several major Health Insurance Companies as an alternative to Medicare. While Managed Care plans may require the insured person to obtain services from someone within a network of service providers, many plans offer superior benefits and access to a broader range of physicians, specialists and surgeons than are available with Medicare.

Issues to consider:

• Is there a specific timeframe for enrollment?

• What doctors can you see?

• What do you have to pay out of pocket?

While people with Medicare may purchase supplemental insurance provided by a separate company, a benefit of a managed care plan is that members often have an option to purchase supplemental coverage as an additional benefit so all coverage is managed by one company. To enroll in a base Medicare HMO plan, there should be no charge as Medicare pays an amount that the HMO accepts as the premium. People that are receiving the Medicare Part B benefit who choose to enroll in a managed care plan continue to pay the monthly Part B premium. The Part B premium is typically deducted from a person's monthly Social Security award payment.

Additionally, many Managed Care Plans provide benefits beyond those that Medicare covers, including such things as preventive care and discounts on prescription drugs, eye care, and the like. Read the descriptions of the managed care plans carefully as they do vary.

Supplemental Insurance

Medicare, like other health insurance plans, does not cover 100% of medical expenses. Instead, only a set amount or percentage is typically covered for approved services. As such, your parent can be responsible for out-of-pocket expenses including deductibles and co-pays beyond the portion covered by Medicare.

To help cover such expenses, many older people find it valuable to have a secondary health care plan – typically referred to as a Medicare Supplement Plan or "Medigap "Insurance.

When considering a Medicare Supplemental Health Care plan, make sure to evaluate the various plans offered. Typically, insurance providers offer a variety of plans that provide the same basic coverage and offer options that may provide for skilled nursing, medical treatment outside your home state, prescription drug coverage options, preventative care options, etc.

While policies vary by state, Medicare supplement insurers, by law, must offer the exact same standard plans so that people can conduct a side-by-side evaluation more easily.   There are 10 standard policies each providing various options in addition to the base coverage. Options include such things as out-of-state coverage, coverage for persons traveling outside the United States, drug benefits, skilled nursing coverage, etc.

Supplemental Plans are typically offered by major Healthcare insurance companies, groups like the AARP and others. When I looked into these plans on behalf of my mother, I was surprised to see that the plans we considered all cost approximately $122 based on her age. People typically have to qualify for these types of plans, therefore someone who is diagnosed with a certain condition (e.g., Alzheimer's) or resides in a certain living environment (e.g., Nursing Home Resident) often times may not qualify.   Therefore, do not wait until the last minute to consider a supplemental insurance plan.

To obtain detailed information about Medigap, I suggest you contact Medicare and request a copy of a government publication entitled: Medicare Supplemental Insurance, Medigap Policies and Protections or Guide to Health Insurance for People with Medicare.

Prescription Drug Considerations

While there has been much hype about the long awaited prescription drug coverage under Medicare, the new drug benefit will not be implemented until 2006. The cost of Prescription drugs is a real issue of many Americans. According to an article from the February 24, 2004 edition of The Cincinnati Enquirer, <u>Poll: Nearly 33% say drug cost a burden</u>. The article indicated that a recent poll by The Associated Press shows approximately one-third of Americans say paying for prescription drugs is a problem in their families. Unfortunately, to avoid the costs, many people reduce their dosages or simply do not receive the medications they need.

In March 2004, the federal government announced the approval of prescription drug cards offered by private firms that will become available in 2004 to people currently on Medicare who do not now have prescription coverage. According to Senator Craig, of the US Senate Special Committee on Aging, *"Medicare officials estimate the temporary drug discount program will save seniors, now without coverage, an estimated 10 to 15 percent on their total drug spending, with discounts of up to 25 percent or more on individual prescriptions. Seniors who have no drug coverage, and whose incomes are below $12,100 a year for an individual or $16,300 per couple, will receive an additional $600 in immediate assistance from the federal government to help them buy the discounted prescriptions. The card providers may charge an annual enrollment fee of up to $30, but there is no enrollment fee for people who qualify for the $600 credit."*

While it may be too early to tell the true value of the newly announced program, there are a number of other programs that are available that may merit investigation. To qualify, many programs have income limitations and require that the applicant not have other prescription drug coverage.

- Prescription Savings Program *(e.g. Together RX)*
- Pharmaceutical Programs *(e.g. Merck Patient Assistance Program)*
- State Sponsored Drug Programs *(e.g. Ohio Golden Buckeye Prescription Drug Savings Program)*
- Pharmacy Programs *(e.g. Walgreen's Dividend Program)*

So how do you find out which program might be best for you? Ask your medical professional, contact your state's Department on Aging, contact the pharmaceutical company that manufacturers your medications, or contact a pharmacy in your area. Ask about savings programs, ways to control and reduce the costs, and how to qualify. Taking the time to research the options that might be available to you and your family could lead to considerable savings.

Medicaid

Many people think that Medicaid and Medicare are two different names for the same program. Actually, they are two different programs. Medicaid is a state-run program designed primarily to help those with low income and little or no financial resources. Medicaid is the national health care assistance program for the poor. Essentially it is a government welfare program. The program is financed by state governments with matching federal funds. Medicaid pays for an estimated 70% of elderly nursing home residents at a cost of more than $50 billion per year. To qualify a person's assets and income must not exceed your state's defined poverty level.

The federal government helps pay for Medicaid, however, each state is responsible for managing its own program including decisions about eligibility requirements and determining what services to cover under Medicaid.

People may consider Medicaid planning because they want their life savings to go to their family and not have their funds depleted paying for long-term care. People with limited assets may consider talking with an attorney that specializes in Medicaid planning to find out if it might make sense to 'shift' assets in order to qualify for Medicaid sooner. Note that Medicaid planning can be risky as the laws are constantly changing and steps that a person takes today may not qualify them in the future.

An article in the November 2003 AARP Bulletin, entitled <u>A New Squeeze on Nursing Home Aid</u> offered some insights on Medicaid. The article indicated that some states, as a result of revenue shortfalls, are asking the Federal government for permission to toughen the Medicaid rules that govern eligibility for nursing home and other health care. To become eligible for Medicaid, *"as the federal law now stands, any gift of cash or property, for example to children, charity, religious organization or political party, made during the three years before applying for Medicaid is considered an improper "transfer of assets" and is subject to a penalty."* Some states want to lengthen the amount of time they can "look back" into an applicant's financial and other records to find these transfers. Currently the 'look-back' period is three years, however, some states want to increase the period to as many as six years.

State governments are trying to avoid people giving away their money and assets today in order get the government to pay for their care tomorrow. Also if a person cannot provide records explaining expenditures, the result could be a denial of coverage.

For more information about the Medicaid program, contact your local medical assistance agency, social service or welfare office.

Cost of Medicine

Do not overlook the cost of medicine. While my sister and I thought that we had our mother's costs covered, there was one we never expected: the cost of her medications. Depending on someone's general health or illness, the monthly cost of medicine can be significant. For our mom, during the last six months of her life, her medicine cost over $1,000 per month.

Earnings Affect Benefits

If your parent is receiving retirement benefits and continues to work, make sure he is aware of the implications. Full retirement age is 65 for people born before 1938 and gradually increases to 67 for people born in 1960 or later. Check with the Social Security Administration and your financial advisor to understand the specific details.

Supplemental Security Income Benefits

Supplemental Security Income (SSI) may be available if your parent has a small income and few assets. If your parent qualifies for Medicaid, food stamps or other assistance, make sure to find out about SSI. As the name implies, Supplemental Security Income "supplements" a person's income up to various levels based on the city and state where he resides. The average SSI for individuals on a monthly basis is $564, whereas for couples the monthly SSI is $846. The federal government pays a basic rate and some states add money to that amount. Check with your local Social Security office for the SSI rates in your state. SSI benefits are financed by general tax revenues and intended to provide minimum monthly income for elderly and disabled persons.

Big Picture Considerations

When dealing with the issues presented in this chapter, you will quickly find that government programs and benefits have wide spread impact on many issues you are likely to encounter.

As our older population expands in the coming years, some experts believe that America's aging population will stretch services to the breaking point. Some states such as Minnesota expect to see the states 60-plus population increase from 16 percent of the population in 2000 to more than 25 percent by 2030. Regardless of the numbers, I have real concern that the costs will rise and our systems will be over capacity.

Summary

As you start to assess and try to understand how Social Security works and the medical benefits your parent is entitled to, people are often disappointed with the monthly award payments and benefits coverage. Also, many people are frustrated by the complexity of the entire system and are challenged by the many interpretations, understanding the caveats, and more. A visit to the Social Security or Medicare website can be frustrating as people are overloaded with information that may not apply to their situation. I suggest that while navigating the system can be challenging in the beginning, once your parent is signed up and receiving his benefits, everything usually goes smoothly.

There is a lot to consider and learn about to ensure your loved one receives all that he is entitled to. Plan ahead; mark key dates in your calendar to ensure you do not miss enrollment dates. Make sure you understand what your loved one is likely to receive so that you are not caught off guard.

In the next chapter I discuss financial matters and look into Long-Term Care insurance. As you understand what is and is not covered by programs such as Medicare, you might want to look into other options that may enable a person to avoid depleting funds when paying for care.

KEY LEARNINGS – *Top three learnings from this chapter:*

1.	
2.	
3.	

ACTION ITEMS - *Things you want to do, or do differently:*

Check when Completed	Action Item	Target Completion Date

9

Estate Matters

The number one concern of elderly people is outliving their assets. This chapter is dedicated to helping you understand estate planning options and to prepare for the future financially. Estate Planning is essentially planning for the management of one's assets during life, and planning for the disposition of one's assets at death. It is suggested that people assess their estate plan annually, or at any time when there is a significant change in one's personal affairs, wealth or property holdings.

Common Questions and Considerations

One of the first questions to consider when thinking about retirement is *"What does your loved one plan to do when he or she retires?" (See Chapter #11 entitled The Talk)* Another common question is *"How much is enough?"* When considering how much is enough, work with a reputable financial advisor or planner to assess your situation. As part of the planning process, make sure to assume a rate of inflation and factor in Social Security benefits. Remember, what might be sufficient to cover annual expenses at age 65, may be inadequate at 80.

Planning for retirement is difficult because everyone is chasing an uncertain and changing target. Money needs to last longer and cover more as a result of people living longer. As family members age, become ill or face injury, loved ones are often forced to make many daunting decisions for which they never planned. Regardless of your situation, it's never to late to consider financial and legal matters.

Everyone has dreams for his or her life and retirement years. The dreams are never to become dependent on someone else for the daily essentials of basic life. Without proper preparation, paying for increased health care or long-term care, especially when it is unexpected, can wipe out a person's lifetime of savings in a few years or even months. So a natural question is *"What can people do now to avoid finding themselves in financial ruin?"* Here are some suggestions:

- Anticipate Assets — Project what you expect to have in terms of assets and cash flow when you retire. Make sure to include Social Security benefits, retirement saving plans, pension plans and survivorship benefits. When tallying your assets, distinguish between 'gross worth' and 'net worth.' Focus on net worth, the amount of cash available after liquidating one's assets and paying taxes and commissions.

- Contemplate Medical History — Based on family health history and personal health, anticipate how long you expect to live, and what type of health-related challenges it might be reasonable to expect.

- Factor In Lifestyle — Give consideration to where you plan to live and the lifestyle you plan to lead. Make sure to factor in a second home, or a move to a different state for a change in climate or to be closer to family.

- Consider Living and Care Arrangements — Assess the various living arrangements and care options paying special attention to cost, personalization of care, and type of care (medical or non-medical / companion). Discuss a loved one's preferences so you are in a position to carry out their wishes at such time as assistance is needed with day-to-day living.

- Project Expenses — Develop your best guess expense budget taking into consideration everyday expenses, projected life expectancy, anticipated changes in lifestyle, liabilities (e.g. outstanding mortgage, car loans and other debt.), and anticipate health-related costs for care, prescription drugs, and more. Also, make sure to factor in travel, new cars and gourmet dining which can be long-denied luxuries that many people treat themselves to in their retirement years.

- Make Changes — Match up the anticipate assets and cash flow with the projected expenses and liabilities to determine at what point in time outliving your assets might become an issue. Make changes as necessary, to either start saving more, or make adjustments to your expected expenses so that you spend less.

Although some experts say most people can retire comfortably and maintain their present standard of living in retirement with about 70-80% of their pre-retirement income, others suggest that a person have savings equal to 20 times their pre-retirement income. While these general recommendations can be a great place to start, savings is only half of the equation.

To know if your savings target is realistic, develop a budget and anticipate your expenses, factor in your projected life expectancy, potential health concerns, care costs, cost of living and lifestyle. Also, make sure to factor in travel, new cars and gourmet dining which can be long-denied luxuries that many people treat themselves to in their retirement years.

One of my favorite quotes about savings was in the client update newsletter I received from my accountant. *"Savings is like exercising. We know we should do it, but many of us give up too quickly because the results are not immediately apparent."* (Source: Sheldon Reder CPA's – Summer 2002)

If you are a caregiver and you have not given much consideraton to your own retirement, there is no better time than now to start. Consider putting aside between 10-20% of your gross income each year. The good news is that cash invested at an 8% interest rate can double in just nine years.

According to the 2003 Retirement Confidence Study, many Americans are seriously unprepared for retirement, either not calculating how much they need to save or underestimating the value of their savings. Planning for retirement is difficult because people are living longer and we are chasing an uncertain and changing target. One thing is for certain; do not rely on Social Security alone as it is not going to be enough for most people to live in the manner to which they are accustom.

As I alluded earlier, don't be surprised if a loved one views money in an entirely different way than you do. Many older people have more of a 'Save' mentality than a 'Spend' mentality. As such, it is not uncommon for an older person's financial values to be focused on saving, frugality and living within one's means. What's most important is having a financial plan, and monitoring and updating the plan to reflect changes.

An insightful article appeared in the December 17, 2002 edition of The Cincinnati Enquirer entitled <u>Retirees' plans hit by losses</u>, written by Brian Tumulty of the Gannett News Service. The article indicated that an AARP survey found that more than three out of four investors age 50 – 70 have lost money over the last two years, with one in five saying the losses will force them to postpone retirement or to work as a retiree.

The point is that things change, people should focus on life, not the daily ups and downs of the stock market. Don't drive yourself crazy each day managing your portfolio, rather, occasionally monitor your financial or estate plans to determine if adjustments should be made to reduce the chance for unexpected surprises. While many older people have a difficult time spending money, it is important for parents not to short change themselves and sacrifice care.

Back to the Basics

While it may seem obvious to many people, I still get questions all the time that indicate people do not have a clear understanding of the term "assets." Assets reflect the total value of a person's accumulated investments and property. Basically, anything that has a cash value (a financial instrument or something that can be sold to raise cash) is considered an asset.

When considering value, be careful. The financial industry uses a terms to reflect wealth that I believe is misleading and incorrect. As part of the retirement planning process, people commonly go through the exercise of tallying their assets to determine their "Net Worth." The only problem is that what is commonly referred to as "Net Worth" is actually "Gross Worth."

People constantly fail to factor in costs associated with liquidating their assets. For example, an IRA is a tax deferred investment, thus, to tap into one's IRA, tax must be paid, drastically reducing the actual value. People also commonly fail to distinguish between insurance value and market value. Whether a sterling silver tea set, a mink coat, car or even a home, the proceeds from the sale of an asset is often much less than expected.

Start with an Inventory

It is important that your parent has an idea of what his estate is worth. To determine someone's worth and cash position, I suggest you begin by completing a detailed inventory of assets. Once that is completed, consider the cash flow your parent will generate on an annual basis including Social Security. Often times, people do not know the items included in a loved one's estate.

There are two options to find out:

1. Encourage, and as appropriate, help a loved one to create an inventory of his or her estate; or

2. Do nothing and be prepared for the treasure hunt of your life.

   (#2 is not recommended)

The logical starting point for many families is to inventory an estate and have a centralized record of everything. Knowing the type of assets that might be available to apply towards one's expenses and care costs can be helpful as families consider living environment and care options.

For most people, documenting the inventory in five categories is sufficient. An explanation of the 'Inventory' process, recommended categories, and suggested level of detail follows:

Suggested Inventory Categories:

1. Transportation	All vehicles leased or owned.
2. Real Estate	All property primary dwelling, time share, commercial property, etc.
3. Home Contents	Contents of the home that may have specific value can be itemized. Other contents may be referred to as a category (e.g., Master Bedroom Suite - $1,000) Make sure to include other notable items such as collectibles, firearms, art, etc.
4. Investments	All types of securities are detailed including 401K, Pension Plans, Annuities, IRA's, etc.
5. Insurance	All insurance plans including Life, Disability, Long-Term Care, etc.

Don't rush through this exercise. The memories shared during the process can have great sentimental value regardless of the financial value a tangible item might have. Take the time to learn when and where certain items were acquired.

Transportation: Under this section list all the forms of transportation that are owned or leased, including auto, motorcycle, boat, all terrain vehicle, RV, pop-up camper, plane, etc. Information you will want to capture and retain includes:

- Vehicle Description
- Make
- Model
- Year
- Name on Vehicle Registration
- Current Monthly Payment
- Current Market Value *(est.)*
- Amount Owed

Don't think that just because it may be Dad's car that it is titled in his name, check the title to be sure. If you're not sure how much a vehicle is worth, look at the classified ads in your local newspaper for a comparable make, model and year, or check with an on-line source such as the Kelley Blue Book at www.kbb.com.

Real Estate: Under this section list all real estate or property including home, condo, vacation property, cabin, time share, land, rental property, commercial building, warehouse space, etc. Details to document include:

- Address
- Brief Description
- Mortgage Company or location of title
- Current Monthly Payment(s)
- Balance Due
- Market Value of Property
- For investment property such as rental housing or commercial space, compile lease agreements, document the names of tenants, monthly rent, etc.

In the case of real estate, it is important to document the name or names for which the property is titled.

Home Contents: Under this section list all home contents either as a category or individually. Home contents include everything from furniture, rugs, antiques, artwork, books, appliances, jewelry, silver, china, etc. It is more important to capture the less obvious or more valuable furnishings than counting four kitchen chairs a toaster, etc. and assigning a value. Instead consider assigning a value to kitchen contents. If there are items on bookshelves that the origin is unknown, such as collectibles, antiques, silverware, and art, make sure to give these items attention.

Don't underestimate the value of something without asking about its history. Something like an old duck decoy or stamp collection could be of significant value.

Investments: This section should include a listing of stocks, bonds, annuities, mutual funds, 401K, IRA, Pension Plans, etc. Details to document include:

- Description of investment (e.g., 10 shares of General Electric Stock)

- Location of Investment Certificates: Is the investment being held in an account, in a safety deposit box, under a mattress, etc. If it is being held somewhere, document the location, account numbers, etc.

- For securities, it may be helpful to document how the investment is titled, designed beneficiaries, # of shares, basis (initial purchase price), and value as of a certain date.

Insurance: List all insurance policies including Life, Disability, Long Term Care, etc. Make sure to capture such policy information as:

- Type
- Cash Value
- Death Benefit
- Named Beneficiary(s)
- Policy Number
- Issuing Company
- Agent/Co. Contact Information

The following exercise is designed to help you assign values to significant assets including autos, home, securities, insurance policies, collectables, and any other notable items of worth. For many families, a parent may want to do this on his own. In cases where your involvement might be seen as an invasion of your parent's privacy, you might consider providing your parent a copy of Exercises #7 and #8 for them to complete. If you do this, be prepared to explain that you are concerned about their future and want to help them determine what financial resources they have available to cover their expenses and care. You can download a more detailed version of this exercise and other exercises from the Aging America Resources website at: www.AgingUSA.com/2004worksheets.asp

EXERCISE #7 – Inventory the Estate		
Transportation (Include cars, boats, RVs, motorcycles, etc.) - Indicate Make, Model & Year	Owner (e.g., Father, Mother or Joint)	NET Market Value (after debts)
	Sub Total	
Home & Contents (Includes residence and notable items of worth (e.g., jewelry, silver, china, guns, collectables, artwork, furnishings, etc.))	Owner	NET Market Value (after mortgage pay-off, sales commissions, etc.)
	Sub Total	
Other Property (Include addresses, tenants and monthly rent, etc.)	Owner	NET Market Value (after mortgage pay-off, sales commissions, etc.)
	Sub Total	
Securities (Stocks, Bonds, IRA, 401K, Pension Plan, etc. Indicate description and location of accounts or actual certificates.)	Provide such detail as number of shares and cost basis (price at time of purchase).	NET Market Value

		Sub Total	
Life Insurance (Indicate name of insurance company, type of insurance and policy number(s))	Estimated Cash Value if surrendered	Estimated Death Benefit
Sub Total		
	TOTAL	

The Treasure Hunt

If your loved one does not plan ahead and inventory his or her estate, it can be up to the family members to try and identify a loved one's assets upon death. If you find yourself completing an inventory without the help of a loved one here are some recommendations that might help you.

1. Start at the bank(s) and inquire about checking and savings accounts.

2. Search safety deposit box or other places where stock certificates, bonds or other securities might be located.

3. Review bank deposits specifically looking for direct deposit dividends.

4. Sift through mail looking for quarterly statements.

5. Refer to recent tax return(s), dividends should be listed as 'Income'. Tax records used to complete a tax return may also provide a lead to a company and broker.

6. Contact former employer(s) to inquire about retirement/pension plans. If a plan was transferred, an employer may be able to locate transfer request, and contact information.

7. Follow-up on Privacy notice(s) received in the US Mail. (Indicates some type of client relationship and may merit a call to inquire.)

Cash Flow

The purpose of the next exercise is to determine the type of cash flow your parent can expect from his investments. When I talk about cash flow, you want to determine the value of dividends, anticipated amount of a required withdrawal from an IRA, and other sources of cash including monthly Social Security award payments.

EXERCISE #8 – Cash Flow		
Detailed Description of income sources (e.g. IRA, 401K, Pension) and Location of Security, Investment or Financial Instruments (e.g., 100 shares of IBM – share certificates in safe deposit box)	Annual Value of Cash Payments Received	Market Value
Totals		

Long-Term Care Insurance

Without proper planning, paying for a long-term care can wipe out a person's lifetime of savings in a few years or even months. According to MetLife, *"on average, people need long-term care for less than 3 years."* In May 2003 the national average cost of a nursing home was approximately $4,800 per month and the national average for a home health aid was approximately $18 per hour.

According to the Health Insurance Association of America, greater than 50% of people age 65 or older are likely to spend some period of time in a nursing home, and an estimated 75% will use formal (paid) care services provided in a home setting. The Wall Street Journal indicated in an article on February 21, 2001, that *"over half of all women and a third of all men 65 and older are expected to spend some time in a nursing home before they die."*

Like auto and home insurance, long-term-care insurance can be a great way to manage risks and avoid financial ruin. The alternatives to LTC insurance are to pay for care out of personal funds, rely on family members for care, or turn to Medicaid (welfare) to cover nursing home stays.

Most insurance coverage provides peace of mind. People pay premiums to protect themselves from loss, with the hope of never having to file a claim. What I find to be intriguing is that older adults have a 1 in 2 chance of incurring a major long-term care expense, yet many people appear to be reluctant to invest in long-term care insurance. While LTC insurance makes financial sense for many people, I believe that people are not ready to believe that they might actually need it.

> *While Aging America Resources does not endorse products or services, I did want to share a brief story that saved our family over $200,000. Shortly after my father passed away, it became very apparent that my mother required on-going care as a result of her dementia. My sister and I were shocked to learn that the communities with specially-designed dementia units cost on average $165 per day. When I was going through my father's records, I found what appeared to be a LTC policy. When I called the insurance company and inquired about the coverage, I was elated to learn that the policy was in force. Apparently, my father had purchased a policy three years earlier and paid an annual premium of approximately $3,000, for three years. While the policy was limited to specific care arrangements and had a maximum daily benefit, it did cover approximately $125 per day for the four plus years that our mother lived in a nursing care facility.*

As people are living longer, the chances increase for someone to encounter unpredictable medical issues that could require long-term treatment or care and be outside the coverage and costs provided by Medicare. Things you might want to think about when considering long-term care insurance include:

- Family health history
- Current 'net' worth and ability to pay for care
- Ability to pay insurance premiums
- Possibility of a surviving spouse requiring care
- Preserving one's estate

In 2001, the LTC insurance industry reportedly paid out more than $1 billion in benefits. LTC policies help pay for health care needs when supervised care is required for extended periods of time. If you consider a policy, find out what type of services are covered. Many older policies cover only nursing homes and in-home care. However, currently available comprehensive policies typically cover an expanded range of services including Assisted Living, Private Duty Nurses, Nurses Aides, Adult Day Care, Homemaker Services, Hospice, and more.

I suggest looking into a number of policies to ensure that you or your loved one gets the best coverage from a reputable provider, and at a competitive price. Do your homework, talk to multiple companies, do a side-by-side comparison, ask family, friends and trusted advisors for referrals, etc. Also, know that people who qualify for Medicaid may not need or have the financial means to pay for LTC insurance.

Long-term policies can be purchased at almost any age. More than half of the LTC policies are reportedly bought by people under age 60. The price of a policy may be drastically lower for someone in his 50's versus someone in his 70's. However, while the monthly premiums may be less for a younger person, since they will likely be paying the premiums for a longer period of time, the policy may end being more expensive. Also, premiums may be subject to increase. If a person waits to secure coverage, he may be more prone to illness or injury that may disqualify a person from receiving coverage. Weigh the options and determine what is best for your situation.

If you choose to evaluate a long-term care policy, you might consider the following questions:

- How much is the annual policy premium? Is the premium payable monthly? Is the premium fixed or subject to change? If it can change, are there limits as to how much or how often?

- If a husband and wife purchase LTC policies is there a discount on the premium? Does the company offer policies with joint coverage that permit both spouses to draw on the total benefit?

- Do any pre-existing conditions disqualify a person from obtaining coverage or receiving benefits? How does the insurer determine if a person is eligible for benefits? Is prior hospitalization required? Does a medical condition need to be diagnosed? Does your parent have to be unable to perform certain day-to-day tasks? Are there certain medical conditions that are NOT covered (e.g. Alzheimer's, addictions)?

- Is there any type of deductible?

- Is the policy renewable for life? Can the policy be cancelled by the company? What happens if a person misses or is late in making a payment?

- What payment options are available? In addition to monthly or annual premiums, some companies offer payment options that enable someone to pay for a policy in full over a shorter period of time (e.g. lump-sum payment, payments over 10 years.)

- Does your parent have to be under the care of a specific person (e.g., RN vs. Nursing Aide)? Do they have to use the services provided by a pre-approved service provider? Is non-medical stand-by assistance covered or does a policy require medical or hands-on assistance?

- Once a person begins to take advantage of the insurance benefit, are premiums still due?

- How does the policy pay out? Amount per day? Does the payout vary by type of care? Is the payout a flat daily amount or is the payout dependent on the actual care expense?

- How is inflation factored into the projected costs? Is there an inflationary adjustment or cost of living adjustment? If benefits are indexed for inflation, is the indexing at simple or compound interest rates?

- Are there any coverage limitations such as requiring a provider to be Medicare certified?

- How does the claims and payment/reimbursement process work? What is the standard turn-around time to pay claims? Are claims paid 30 days in arrears?

- Once you have a need to take advantage of the coverage, how long of a period (often referred to as a waiting period) is there before the policy starts to pay out? Often policies can have waiting periods from one month to one-year. What are the options? How are the premiums different? How does the waiting period work?

- What other options might be available that could further reduce the cost of the premiums? (e.g., purchase through an organization or group plan, husband and wife buying plans at the same time and receiving a marital discount, etc.)

- If the LTC insurance company has made enhancements to the policy offerings, are enhancements available to existing policy owners? Will additional charges apply?

- Are the policy benefits taxable as income or tax exempt? Qualified policy benefits are received tax free, where as non-qualified policies are generally taxable to the insured as benefits are paid.

Long-term care benefits can often be paid directly to the care provider organization by completing an Assignment of Benefits form. These forms, along with an Authorization of Medical Information form, must be renewed annually by the person receiving the benefit or by someone with Power of Attorney.

Price should not be the primary basis for a buying decision as rates are not guaranteed. Also, make sure to consider the financial solvency of the provider company. With the benefit payouts exceeding $1 billion a year, make sure you are with a provider that is reputable and stable. You may want to check with the Better Business Bureau and/or State's Insurance Department to discover what type of complaints, if any, have been filed against a particular provider.

Another option that is available through many larger employers is buying LTC coverage as part of your employee benefits package. Coverage may be available to employees for themselves, a spouse, parents or in-laws. Benefits of group coverage as opposed to individual coverage often includes lower premiums and plans may be easier to qualify as there are often fewer health questions. If you consider a group policy, make sure to understand your options to maintain coverage if you leave the company (e.g. resignation, termination, separation, retirement.)

Life Insurance
If you or a loved one has any type of life insurance (e.g., term, variable) make sure the beneficiary designations are up-to-date. As I indicated in Chapter #7 – Legal Planning, proceeds from insurance pass directly to the beneficiaries upon death and are not subject to a Will or Trust. In the case of a divorce or remarriage or death of a beneficiary, make sure to update the beneficiary information in your policies.

Many life insurance policies have a cash value in addition to a death benefit. Speak with your insurance agent to find out the specifics of your policy and how you may be able to draw against the cash value should you find yourself needing cash. Also, inquire as to when a policy may expire and what options might be available to continue coverage.

Estate and Death Taxes
While the federal estate tax is being phased out over a number of years, it remains uncertain if the tax will be repealed and become permanent. An estate is exempt from federal estate taxes if it's below the following thresholds:

2004 - 2005 - $1.5 million

2006 - 2008 - $2.0 million

2009 - $3.5 million

2010 - No tax

2011 - To Be Determined

Regardless of what happens on the federal level, many states impose death taxes. States are imposing death taxes in part to replace revenues lost by the declining federal estate tax. States with death tax include: Connecticut, District of Columbia, Illinois, Indiana, Iowa, Kansas, Kentucky, Louisiana, Maine, Maryland, Massachusetts, Minnesota, Nebraska, New Jersey, New York, North Carolina, Ohio, Oklahoma, Oregon, Pennsylvania, Tennessee, Vermont, Virginia, Washington and Wisconsin. Check with your legal or financial advisor for the most current information specific to your state.

Annual Exclusions and Gifting

People with sizable estates might find it appropriate to share their wealth in a way that is tax-free. People can make annual gifts of $11,000 to family, friends and charitable organizations (other than employees) they wish without any estate tax consequences. When might this be appropriate? If the size of someone's estate is in excess of the Applicable Exclusion (the amount that is not subject to estate tax upon death).

In the above example, I focus on making gifts if the value of an estate is in excess of the then current estate tax exclusion amount. Is that the only time your parent might want to gift? Speak with your parent and his or her legal and financial advisors to discuss your family's specific situation and determine if gifting might be appropriate.

At any time in your parent's life, she can pass along an amount up to or equal to the then current estate tax exclusion amount without any estate tax consequences. That could be a single payout of $1.5 million, three payouts of $500,000, or any other combination – not to exceed the exemption amount. Benefits of distributing money to children during a parent's lifetime include: To help kids establish their lives, to help them with home or education expenses, to pay off loans, to provide a nest egg for their grandkids' education, to transfer the money so that the kids and even grandkids could get the benefit of the appreciation of the money.

Depending on his wishes, a parent may choose to transfer funds to a Trust established for children and/or grandchildren so that he has some say in how the money is used, when it becomes available, etc. Again, speak with your legal or financial advisor to discuss your situation.

> *If a loved one is considering making a gift of appreciated stocks to family, it may be worth a quick analysis. If the cost basis (original purchase price) was $5,000 and if the stock is now valued at $10,000, tax would be due on the $5,000 capital gain. To keep this example simple, assume the person is in the 30% tax bracket. That would mean that the $10,000 gift only generated $8,500 of cash value because $1,500 or 30% of the $5,000 appreciated value is payable as tax. Therefore I suggest that if a parent's estate can afford to pay the tax consequence without over diluting her remaining assets, the parent might sell the stock and transfer cash so the recipient receives the benefit of the entire $10,000 gift.*

Since the laws regarding lifetime exclusions and gifting are still being assessed and reassessed I suggest, wherever possible, making reference to the authority being granted in the POA without referring to currently approved dollar amounts. In other words, today a person can gift $11,000 annually. If the allowable amount for tax free gifts increases to $15,000, a person's authority to gift would be limited if $11,000 was indicated in the POA. Therefore I suggest language such as *"authorization to annually make gifts at the maximum allowable tax free amount."*

Reverse Mortgages

Reverse mortgages enable a home owner to convert home equity into cash. Money received from a reverse mortgage is tax-free. There is typically a closing cost associated with initiating a reverse mortgage. Reverse mortgages enable people age 62 and older to borrow against their home's value without having to repay the loan during their lifetime. The amount borrowed including accrued interest, can't exceed the value of a person's home. According to an article in the April 19, 2004 edition of Business Week, *"tighter budgets among U.S. seniors and greater consumer awareness are fueling a boom in reverse mortgages."*

Reverse mortgages provide a way for people who need cash to cover their expenses. With a reverse mortgage, a person either uses it to stop making monthly mortgage payments or to receive a flat monthly payout. Reverse mortgages can also provide a way for people to pay for either LTC insurance or long-term care.

In addition to reverse mortgages, there are a number of other ways to get money out a person's home. One option is opening a line of credit. With a line of credit, a person takes a loan against the principle of the home and makes monthly payments to repay the loan. The two primary differences are the loan is a lump-sum amount as opposed to being a set monthly amount. Also, with a line of credit, there is an expectation to pay back the loan on a monthly basis. Another option that many people consider is to downsize to a smaller home enabling a person to free up home equity and potentially reduce operating costs.

There are a number of types of reverse mortgages that vary in regards to closing costs, insurance requirements, interest rates, and the percentage of home value that can be mortgaged. If you or a loved one considers a reverse mortgage, make sure to consider a number of options and mortgage companies. Since Reverse mortgages are not something that most people are familiar with, I encourage you to take the time and read the fine print. For more information on reverse mortgages, contact the National Reverse Mortgage Lender's Association at www.reversemortgage.org.

Charitable Giving

While I made references to Trust documents in Chapter #7 – Legal Planning, many people, especially those with sizable estates, may wish to consider charitable giving options. Gifts can be restricted for a specific purpose or gifts can be unrestricted giving the beneficiary organization total control over the funds for whatever endeavors or projects it sees fit. Gifts can be made during a person's lifetime as well as upon death. Also, there are a number of options available to people from gifting proceeds for life insurance, gifting appreciated securities, cash and more. The following is a summary of the options that may be available to people:

- CASH GIFT – gifting cash during a person's lifetime provides an immediate tax benefit to the person making the gift and provides the charitable organization with funds for current use. When making a cash gift, make sure that the gift is in fact tax deductible and that the organization can provide you with the necessary information for tax purposes.

- APPRECIATED SECURITIES – many people have securities (e.g. stocks) that have appreciated considerably over the years. Gifting appreciated stocks can be advantageous because there is no capital gains tax when the actual shares are transferred and the recipient of the gift benefits from the entire amount of the gift. For tax purposes, the person making a gift can claim the full market value of the securities calculated on the date the gift was transferred.

- CHARITABLE REMAINDER TRUST – The name suggests how this tool works.
  - Charitable - the basic purpose of the trust is to leave money to a charity.
  - Remainder - the designated charity or charities gets the remainder, or what is left after a person dies.
  - Trust – when you set-up a trust, you no longer own the property or money you put in it – the trust does.

  CRT's are often desirable to people who wish to make a gift to one or more charities, often of appreciate stock, and also want to maintain a stream of income during their life. A percentage of the ongoing value or a fixed dollar amount is paid to an income beneficiary during their life. What remains in the trust, no less than 10%, is payable to one or more charities upon death. A CRT is an irrevocable trust. In other words once you place assets in the trust, you can not get them back out and decide to use them in a different way. You can name yourself trustee and decide how the money is invested. The money the charity gets is not subject to estate taxes.

- FAMILY FOUNDATIONS – can be an effective way for individuals with a high net worth to support charities or other philanthropic causes while minimizing tax consequences on their wealth. A family foundation is considered a charitable organization. For more information, contact your financial advisor.

Retiree Benefits

Many companies that may have offered health insurance and other benefits for life are reducing or eliminating benefits. Many plans are under funded as they did not expect the increases to health care and related care costs. If your loved one is counting on company benefits after retirement, find out what coverage is guaranteed and what happens in the case of bankruptcy, merger or acquisition.

An article in the February 13, 2003 edition of The Cincinnati Enquirer entitled <u>Retirees losing health benefits,</u> indicated that thousands of retired workers who were promised life-time health care coverage by their former companies have lost those benefits as a growing list of firms have folded or been sold.

The following is from an article written by John Eckberg that was featured in the February 10, 2004 edition of The Cincinnati Enquirer entitled <u>Is your pension fund secure?</u> *"Generally, pension benefits are not at risk when a company declares bankruptcy because the pension assets must be kept in a separate account from other company operating funds. The funds are usually held in trust or invested in an all-insurance contract, according to the US Dept. of Labor's employee benefits security administration."* ...But that doesn't mean that the company hasn't funded the plan poorly. The federal Pension Benefit Guaranty Corporation assumes responsibility when problems occur.

Other Financial Considerations

- Hire Someone to Handle Finances - Many older people may not be comfortable handling their personal finances, especially in the case of a surviving spouse that has not been involved in day-to-day financial decisions and bill paying. An emerging profession is what is referred to as money managers. Money managers are people who handle bill paying and organizing records for tax purposes. Older adults may not want to burden their kids or frankly may not trust their kids. If you consider a money manager, make sure the individual is bonded and insured. Money managers typically charge between $35 - $85 an hour.

- Claiming Parents as Dependents – According to the Financial Planning Association, there may be tax breaks for people who are financially supporting their aging parents. To qualify, a person must provide more than half of the person's support for the tax year. Support includes paying for food, shelter, clothing, medical expenses, and more. There are also income requirements for a person to be claimed as a dependent. Contact a tax specialist to determine what you might be entitled to claim and deduct.

- Minimizing Tax Consequences – Many investment options can help people shield retirement savings from taxes. Discuss tax deferred or tax-free investment opportunities with your financial planner. Popular options include:
  - 401(k) and 403(b) plans – contributions aren't taxed, but you pay income taxes on withdrawals.
  - Roth IRA – you can't deduct your contributions, but gains are not taxed and withdrawals are tax-free.

Big Picture Considerations

Getting involved with someone's personal finances can be awkward and uncomfortable. Unfortunately, the majority of people have not planned well. If a parent is having a difficult time making ends meet, you may feel guilty as you determine what or how much to help without compromising your own financial position and ability to provide for your family. There can be so many unexpected expenses, especially for people who face any type of illness. The cost of medical care can wipe out a person's finances in a short period of time.

If you find that your parent has insufficient resources to provide for a desired or needed level of care, consider the possible merits of shifting assets in order to qualify for Medicaid. Before you would consider anything as drastic as trying to qualify for Medicaid, make sure to seek professional advice from your family attorney and financial planner. Everyone involved should understand the type of care environment that would be provided by Medicaid.

If you are named in a loved one's Will and receive inheritance, I caution you not to make any drastic life changes during the first year after a parent's death. Just as when people get a raise at work, few end up having the extra money available to enjoy. The same can happen for inheritance. I know of many people who have acted irresponsibly with inheritance, changed their lifestyle and then found themselves relying solely on their own income as any savings (inheritance) was spent. If you are fortunate enough to be named in your loved one's Will to receive inheritance, be careful and act responsibly. Most people find that there are plenty of raining days ahead and wish they would have saved for a rainy day.

192

Summary

While there may be many financial tools and options available to people, financial issues tend to be quite personal. While I have provided an overview of the many considerations and alternatives, I suggest you work with a professional in the financial industry to determine which options and strategies may make the most sense for your particular situation. Recognize that the industry term of Net Worth isn't actually net worth and plan accordingly. Make sure to anticipate expenses and establish a budget based on life expectancy and potential health concerns and care needs.

Make sure to maintain an up-to-date inventory of all personal property and make sure you and your loved ones understand the concept of assets and gross worth. Remember, it is never too late to start saving.

KEY LEARNINGS – *Top three learnings from this chapter:*
1.
2.
3.

ACTION ITEMS - *Things you want to do, or do differently:*		
Check when Completed	*Action Item*	*Target Completion Date*

10

End-Of-Life Planning

This chapter addresses end-of-life care, funeral considerations and specific things families can do to prepare and plan for death. While death may be a taboo subject for many people, it is a reality for all people. As Ben Franklin is quoted as saying, *"Two things in life a certain – death and taxes."*

I am surprised that more people don't do end-of-life or memorial planning. Many people I talk with suggest that planning will result in a sooner death. The analogy I offer has to do with people watching their favorite sports team on television. Some people believe that every time they turn on the TV to watch their favorite sports team compete, they lose. Therefore, if they don't watch the game, the team will win. Just as sports teams will win or lose regardless if a particular person is watching or not, a person's death is not going to occur sooner or later as a result of planning or failing to plan.

According to the National Center for Health Statistics and the Population Division, approximately 7,000 people die daily or 2.4 million annually. That is equal to roughly 1% of the U.S. population. A far greater number of people find themselves facing illness, injury or disease on any given day that could turn their lives upside down.

Decision Support Tools
If you or a loved one is facing tough decisions, you might want to investigate one or more of the following web-based tools that are designed to help families make life and death treatment decisions. According to an article in the October 10, 2002 edition of The Wall Street Journal, many of the tools are *"Great for "validation." In other words, the tools can give people confidence in the treatment plan his doctor recommends and also learned more about*

other options." I believe that there is a natural tendency for families to seek out information and be confident that they are not only doing the right things, but, that they are also doing all the things they could or should.

One decision support tool is the Heart Profiler available from the American Heart Association (www.AmericanHeart.org.) The profiler is a personalized online tool that people can use to understand their risks and make life-and-death treatment decisions. Other treatment decision tools or health decision guides are available from such website as www.Cancer.org, www.MayoClinic.com and www.MerckSource.com.

Whether using the Heart Profiler or any other on-line profile type tool, be careful. Many web-based profilers have some sort of sponsorship from drug companies, clinical trial recruiters and other companies with a marketing agenda that patients should be aware of before participating. Also, using any type of on-line tool should not be considered a substitute for consulting with a medical professional about a particular illness or concern.

Palliative or Hospice Care

One decision that many families face is when to switch from curative treatments to palliative care. An article from the April 14, 2003 edition of the USA Today entitled <u>The Courage to face the end</u>, offers some interesting insight. *"Palliative care focuses on life, not illness." "Palliative care focuses on reducing discomfort or suffering and improving quality of life so people can live life to the fullest...Palliative Care doesn't mean you make a decision and forego any future treatments. You still need to assess the situation and options as they arise...If she's focusing on the illness, she's not focusing on life."*

Hospice is a philosophy that focuses on comfort care as opposed to cure. Hospice staff and volunteers work with family members to plan and manage a loved one's care. Hospice care may include physical and occupational therapy, speech/language pathology services, dietary and other counseling, intravenous fluids, and other care to help a person maintain comfort. Services also include arranging for equipment, supplies, and medicines.

So how is Curative and Palliative Care different? Curative care emphasizes the use of medicine and medical procedures to cure or control disease. According to www.HospiceWeb.com, *"Hospice (Palliative) care is a choice you make to enhance life for a dying person. A person with a terminal disease may choose to die at home with the support of family, friends, and caring professionals. Hospice care emphasizes comfort measures and counseling to provide social, spiritual and physical support to the dying patient and his or her family. All hospice care is under professional medical supervision."* Over 90% of hospice care is provided in the patient's home, according to information posted on the website.

The November 19, 2003 edition of The Loveland Herald featured an article by guest columnist Chaplin Darin Lewis. In the article he stated that Hospice is often associated with Death – a place where one goes to die. *"Hospice isn't a place where one goes to die; it's a place where one goes to live." "We're not here to hasten death. We're here to make people comfortable. It doesn't mean the individual has given up. It just means that they have resolved themselves to the fact that they know this disease is going to end up taking their life. They just want to have time to really live before they die."*

Hospice care is often viewed as synonymous with the inevitable death and the unavailability of curative treatment. An article in the February 2003 Journal of American Geriatrics Society (JAGS), entitled <u>Care of Patients Near Death, Another View</u>, by Elizabeth Steel and Jill Kulbe, offered what I believe to be a wonderful, but not so common, way to think of hospice. *"One Dr. recommends thinking about it as Plan A and Plan B. Plan B is the back-up plan to Plan A, a curative treatment. This manner of presentation appears to have the following benefits. First, the patient can continue to hope for the development of a curative treatment (Plan A) and can then discontinue Hospice. Second, the patient can maintain the sense of "fighting" that is so often important. Third, the fear of impending death is muted. Finally, the patient will be cared for compassionately throughout the course of the illness."*

Let me clear up a misnomer. Hospice is not a place. Hospice services can be provided in a number of settings including a person's home, a hospice center, and a hospital.

According to Medicare, there are four levels of hospice care, which are paid for by Medicare, Medicaid and most other insurance plans. Some or all of these care options may be used when a patient receives hospice care.

1. **Routine Care**: The patient lives and receives care at home. The family and patient are able to handle the needs and care of the patient with assistance from the hospice team.

2. **Continuous Care**: Skilled nursing services are provided in the patient's home to help manage a patient's symptoms.

3. **Inpatient Care**: Inpatient care is provided for a limited period of time in a hospital, nursing home, or other care facility for symptoms or crises that cannot be managed in the patient's home.

4. **Respite Care**: Respite care provided in a facility and is designed to give caregivers a rest from their caregiver responsibilities. Respite care is limited to five days and nights at a time.

The hospice or the attending physician determines the appropriate level of care.

Medicare Hospice Benefits

Hospice Care is provided in 60 or 90 day periods of care. At the start of each period, the attending physician must certify that a person is terminally ill and probably has less than six months to live. If a person qualifies for Hospice, he or she will receive medical and support services covered by Medicare. Hospice Care is covered under Medicare Part A – Hospital Insurance. To receive benefits, care must be provided from a Medicare-approved hospice program.

WHAT'S COVERED?
- Physician Services
- Nursing Care
- Medical Equipment (such as wheelchairs and walkers)
- Medical Supplies (such as bandages and catheters)
- Drugs for symptom control and pain relief
- Short term care in the hospital, including respite care
- Home health aide and homemaker services
- Physical and occupational therapy
- Speech therapy
- Social worker services
- Dietary counseling
- Counseling to help you and your family with grief and loss

WHAT'S NOT COVERED?
- Treatment to cure a terminal illness
- Room and board (e.g. home/nursing home)

For more information on Hospice and Palliative Care or to find a hospice program in your area, visit one of the following organizations listed below or refer to your local Yellow Pages telephone directory:

- The National Hospice Organization – www.nho.org, 800-658-8898

- The Hospice Association of America – www.hospice-america.org, 202-546-4759

- The National Hospice and Palliative Care Organization – www.nhpco.org, 703/837-1500

There may be many different providers of Hospice Care in your area. As with any care arrangement, I suggest you give careful consideration when selecting a Hospice Program. Specific things you might ask about include the following:

- What is your process for understanding and honoring a care recipient's wishes?

- How is pain assessed and managed on an on-going basis?

- What is the preferred care setting? Are certain settings required to manage crisis situations?

- Is the Hospice Medicare and Medicaid certified?

- What type of training and support services are available to family members?

- What type of working arrangements are there between a person's current physician or medical team and the Hospice physician and staff?

- What type of care coverage and attention should a family expect (e.g. frequency and duration of care)? What are the standard hours of care? How is after-hours care handled?

- How are staff assignments made? How many care recipients are assigned to a lead staff person?

- What type of staff experience, qualifications or training should be expected? What staff, if any, is volunteer?

- What staff expertise should a family expect to be part of a care team?

- What might a typical day of Hospice care entail?

Funeral Considerations

Many decisions need to be made specific to a loved one's remains and final disposition. Additionally, there is a lot to consider when planning a funeral or memorial service. The type of funeral decisions people need to make include the following:

- Funeral Home of choice
- Pre-Arrange, Pre-Paid or neither
- Place of Funeral – Church, Synagogue, Funeral Home, etc.
- Method of Interment or Final Disposition (e.g. Burial, Cremation, Entombment, Mausoleum)
- Name and Location of Cemetery and Plot
- Location of Deed to Cemetery Plot
- Person to Officiate (e.g. Pastor, Rabbi)
- Pall Bearers
- Particular Wishes for the actual ceremony
- Memorial Giving

Pre-Planned Funerals

There are many different terms used to refer to funeral planning including Pre-Arranged, Pre-Planned, Pre-Funded and Pre-Paid. Let me begin with a review of these terms.

- PRE-PLANNING, Pre-Need Planning and Pre-Arrangement are interchangeable terms that mean a person is handling their own memorial planning so that loved ones don't have to make difficult decisions. An increasing number of people (*including the late President Ronald Reagan*) are choosing to pre-arrange their funeral to reduce pressure and uncertainty when a death occurs. People often think of pre-arrangement as part of the estate planning process where choices are thoroughly considered and decisions are made. Advance planning involves making selections regarding the funeral home, disposition of a body, casket selection, burial plot, visitation or viewing, the obituary, and funeral considerations such as song choices, readings, the person to preside over the ceremony and more. If a loved one pre-arranges a funeral, make sure someone knows where the instructions are located so family members can access the document. Pre-Arrangement is not the same as Pre-Paid. A person can specify all the arrangements, however, the specific services may not be paid for until a death occurs and services are rendered.

- PRE-PAID and Pre-Funded are terms that involve paying for services in advance of need. In order to pre-pay for services, a person must make selections and pre-arrange their funeral. When a person pays for services in advance, he or she enters into what is referred to as a Pre-Need Contract. The contact stipulates the specific products and services that are part of the contractual arrangement. If a loved one pre-pays for a funeral, make sure that a receipt is on-file with the arrangement instructions so that your family does not unnecessarily pay or make arrangements with a different provider. It is estimated that as many as 1/3rd of all funerals in the U.S. are paid for in advance.

In most states, the money that is paid in advance for the contractual arrangements is required by law to be placed in a separate trust account and the funds may only be used for their specific purpose. Additionally, a funeral home is supposed to provide an accounting to the state of all funds each year and protect the money by maintaining a bond. If you or a member of your family considers pre-paying for funeral, ask what happens if the funeral home is sold or goes out of business. Also, inquire what happens if a person moves to a different city or state. Is the prepaid amount refundable?

Themed Funerals

While people often think of funerals as being rather somber, many people are choosing to remember loved ones with a themed celebration. According to an article in the December 16, 2002 edition of Business Week, *"Undertakers are reporting a boom in themed funerals."* For a themed funeral, the décor and the celebration is centered around a personal passion such hunting, cooking, or even a favorite sports teams. According the article, the NFDA, indicates that as many as half the funerals now have themes with family members and friends providing the props.

Embalming

Because the human body begins to decompose as soon as death occurs, funeral directors and their staff help maintain or preserve a body by embalming the deceased. The process includes a thorough cleansing using chemicals and other practices that will preserve and restore a body for a temporary period. Embalming allows a body to be laid out for a visitation or memorial service. Family and friends have a final chance to say their good-byes and validate the loss by viewing their loved one. This often helps confirm the reality of death. Embalming can be a personal preference, basis of religious belief or ethnicity.

Cremation

The Cremation Association of North America (CANA) projects by 2025, more than half of all people who die in the US will be cremated. In 2000, over 600,000 people, approximately 26% of deaths, had remains cremated. When a person's remains are cremated, the ashes from the cremation are collected and placed in a sealed container the size of a small box approximately 4x4x4 and weighing approximately 5-10 pounds.

Cremation is often a personal preference; however, cremation may also be the choice based on religious preference or ethnicity. When a body is to be cremated, the funeral director must apply for permits from the local health department. In many states there is a waiting period before a body can be cremated, since the cremation itself would prohibit any further medical examination, such as cause-of-death or DNA identification.

People often have special wishes for the final disposition of their ashes. While cremains are often buried in an urn on a cemetery plot, we have all heard the stories of people who want their ashes spread on a football field, in the ocean, or some other special place. If it is your intention to scatter the ashes, your funeral director can advise of any local or state regulations.

Funeral and Related Costs

Federal Law requires that funeral directors provide an itemized list of prices to families. Families have the right to pick and chose services as they wish. While packages may offer price incentives, a funeral provider can not require a family to purchase a package. A funeral home cannot refuse, or charge a handling fee for, a casket purchased elsewhere and provided by the family. For information on funeral rules and requirements, or to request a free publication entitled Funerals: A Consumer Guide, contact the Federal Trade Commission. The Consumer Guide is available on-line at www.ftc.gov/bcp/conline/pubs/service/funeral.pdf.

End-Of-Life Planning

The average cost of a funeral is over $5,000. While there are many options and possible charges associated with a funeral, some of the standard services and typical price range are as follows. Packages are often available that provide a lower price when multiple services are purchased. Also, the prices vary by city and state. Make sure to request a General Price List from the funeral home of your choice in advance of making preparations so you are aware of the various services offered and associated charges.

Professional service charge	$1,250 - $1,500
Transfer of Body to Funeral Home	$150 - $250
Embalming	$500 - $600
Preparation of Remains for Viewing	$150 - $250
Visitation	$350 - $500
Funeral at Funeral Home	$400 - $500
Honorarium for Person Officiating Funeral	$100 - $500
Honorarium for Vocalist/Musician	$75 - $150
Cremation	$400 - $450
Hearse	$200 - $300
Service Car / Van	$75 - $100
Limousine	$200 - $300
Casket	$500 - $10,000

An article in the February 2, 2004 edition of Business Week entitled Double Wide Nation indicated that nearly one-third of Americans are obese. If a standard size casket does not accommodate a loved one, larger size caskets, up to triple wides are available through Goliath Casket.

Charges may also be associated with running a classified obituary in the newspaper, obtaining certified copies of the death certificate, flowers, burial container, burial vault or container. Additional charges separate from the Funeral Home services include cemetery expenses and the cost of a headstone or monument. Grave markers can take months to complete and can be expensive. Pricing and delivery is determined by the type of stone chosen, size and wording. Your funeral director can make a recommendation on a company to handle the gravestone. The company that provides the gravestone will coordinate the delivery and installation with the cemetery. Note that gravestones are not just offered at earth burials. Gravestones are also placed on top of an urn of ashes and even used as a marker for remembrance purposes when a loved one's ashes are not present.

Funeral Payment Options

When a person pre-arranges and pre-pays for a funeral, the cost is determined by the general price list that is in effect at the time the contract is executed. If a person pre-arranges, but does not pre-pay, the pricing of products and services is based on the general price list in effect at the time of death.

In addition to executing a Pre-Need Contract, there are others ways for people and families to pay for funeral services. A life insurance policy may be purchased for final expenses with a benefit that is expected to be equal to or greater than the cost of the funeral. Second, establish a savings account or other financial instrument (certificate of deposit) that is designated for funeral expenses, and the funds are payable on death to a funeral home. A third option is to pay for the cost of a funeral with funds from a person's estate.

If a parent or loved one served our country in the Armed Forces, he or she may be eligible for special benefits and a burial allowance. Contact the Veteran's Benefit Administration at 800-827-1000 or visit them on-line at www.cem.va.gov/benvba.htm.

When a person dies, there is a one-time Government Benefit, paid through Social Security in the amount of $255 that can be applied to funeral expenses. Also, if your loved one has limited financial resources, he or she might be eligible for assistance with funeral costs from Medicaid. Contact Medicaid for information and eligibility requirements.

The Obituary

While everyone has seen obituaries in a local newspaper, most people do not understand how the process works and what charges apply. There are two different kinds of obituaries, Classified Obituaries and Editorial Obituaries:

- Classified Obituaries are paid for on a line-by-line basis similar to a standard classified advertisement.

- Editorial Obituaries are stories typically written by the news staff at the local newspaper.

End-Of-Life Planning

Classified obituaries often focus on basic information about a person, surviving family members and information about the funeral arrangements. For example,

- John Doe, beloved husband of Jane Doe (nee Maiden Name), dear father of (insert names), brother of (Insert Names), died (Insert date) at Age (Insert age). Also survived by many nieces, nephews and grandchildren. Indicate arrangements. Indicate Memorials may be made to (Insert Name and Address of Organization).

Beside the basic information, people often like to include additional information about a loved one's military service, work history, professional achievements, community contributions and more. For example,

- John Doe, beloved husband of Jane Doe (nee Maiden Name), dear father of (insert names), brother of (Insert Names), died (Insert date) at Age (Insert age). Also survived by many nieces, nephews and grandchildren. ADD any Military service, Graduated from (Insert name of School), was employed as (Job Title) at (Name of Company) for (Insert Number of Years) before retiring in (Insert Year). Actively involved in (Name of Organization). EXPAND any of the information above and ADD any memberships to clubs or organizations, Personal and Professional Achievements. Indicate arrangements. Indicate Memorials may be made to (Insert Name and Address of Organization).

Other obituary considerations include:
- Indicate any other residences. (John, a resident of Bradenton, Florida, since his retirement in 1995...)
- Indicate that in lieu of flowers, memorial contributions may be sent to _____ (if this is your desire).
- Decide if you will include a photo of the deceased.

Editorial obituaries often feature prominent citizens, community leaders and people who have served our great country. The challenge with an editorial obituary is that there is no guarantee of placement. If you believe your loved one's life and contributions merits an editorial obituary, ask your funeral director for the name and number of the person at the local newspaper who writes the obituaries. Then call that person to verify his or her expectations and learn what information he or she may need. Request a fax number and e-mail so you can send information. I suggest you be prepared to provide the following information:

- Name
- Age
- Residence
- Information on spouse (living or dead)
- Educational background
- Community and personal interests and involvement
- Work history
- Professional achievements
- Community contributions
- Affiliation with local clubs and organizations
- Date, time and location of memorial service
- Organization name for honorariums
- Contact name and number for additional information

Know that there is no guarantee an Editorial Obituary will run. I have heard stories of prominent citizens and decorated war veterans whose stories never ran because a human interest obituary was run instead. The point is, unless you are a local celebrity, you may be better off not expecting anything and being happily surprised if a story runs.

A Tribute and an Example

The following are my parents' obituaries that appeared in the Metro section of our local daily newspaper:

Obituaries – *March 3, 1997*

Charles G. Puchta, 79, was lawyer, civic leader
Posts included presidency of chamber of commerce

By William A. Weathers
The Cincinnati Enquirer

Charles G. Puchta, retired senior partner with Cincinnati's Frost & Jacobs Law firm and a civic activist, died Sunday in Jewish Hospital. Mr Puchta, of Hyde Park, was 79. His community activities included serving as president of the Greater Cincinnati Chamber of Commerce. During his tenure, he led the chamber's first trade mission to Japan in 1978.

Mr. Puchta joined Frost & Jacobs in 1943 after receiving a degree from the University of Cincinnati College of Law. A native of Cincinnati and a 1936 graduate of Walnut Hills High School, he received a bachelor's from UC in 1940.

When he retired in November after 53 years with the law firm, colleague John S. Stith said, "More than anyone else, Charlie made certain that we all learned that the practice of law is a profession, but the administration of a law firm is a business. In terms of financial success of the firm that leadership without doubt permitted Frost & Jacobs to make several quantum leaps. Charlie pushed to professionalize our administrative staff and to move into the ear of greater productivity through technology."

Puchta devoted much of his spare time to charitable and civic activities. In 1992, the Greater Cincinnati chapter of the Juvenile Diabetes Foundation honored him as its Cincinnatian of the Year. Mr Puchta was humble when he accepted the award, saying it was "truly a great honor for me. Quite frankly, I'd have been delighted to the Cincinnatian of the month – even for a short month like February."

He also was former board chairman of the Cincinnati Nature Center and trustee of the UC Foundation. Mr. Puchta served Hebrew Union College through his chairmanship of the executive committee for its annual Associates Tribute Dinners. He also was chairman of the 1976 Mobilized for Xavier University Campaign and a co-founder of the Father O'Connor Club at Xavier. Most recently, Mr. Puchta has served on the board of trustees of Jewish Hospital.

"Charlie provided a great deal of leadership on the board...for the last eight years," hospital President Warren Falberg said Sunday. "It was a time of a lot of change for the hospital and provided significant leadership."

Said is son, Charles Jr. of Symmes township: "He did love charitable and civic-type activities. It was more of a privilege than a business duty." Other survivors include his wife Jean; his daughter Polly Wells of Mariemont; and four grandchildren.

A memorial service will be 11 a.m. Wednesday in Armstrong Chapel, 5125 Drake Road in Indian Hill. There will be no visitation. The body will be cremated. Contributions can be made to the Juvenile Diabetes Foundation, 10901 Reed Hartman Highway, Blue Ash, 45242.

Obituaries - November 27, 2001

Jean G. Puchta, 70, taught school, Braille

She was also devoted to her church's choir

By Rebecca Billman
The Cincinnati Enquirer

GREENHILLS -- Jean G. Puchta, a former fourth-grade teacher at Cincinnati Country Day School, died Saturday at the Alois Alzheimer Center, where she lived for the past three years.

A certified Braillist, Mrs. Puchta, 70, also worked with the Junior League and the National Council of Jewish Women, typing Braille materials and teaching Braille to students enrolled in Cincinnati Public Schools, according to her son, Charles Puchta Jr. of Symmes Township. She was a fun-loving person who "could talk anybody's ear off," her son said. "She was a wonderful advocate for things she believed in and loved." One of those things was church music. A member of the Indian Hill Episcopal-Presbyterian Church choir, she led the group on a choral mission trip to England.

Mrs. Puchta moved to Cincinnati from Boston to accept the position at Cincinnati Country Day in the 1950s. A native of Pelham Manor, N.Y., she received a bachelor's degree in philosophy and religion from Wheaton College in Norton, Mass., and a master's degree in elementary education from Harvard University. Before moving here, she taught at the Newington Home and Hospital in Hartford, Conn., and on the polio floor of Children's Hospital in Boston.

She was a member of the Cincinnati Women's Club and on the board of the Cincinnati branch of the English-Speaking Union, a nonprofit organization that promotes scholarship and the effective use of English in the global community. She was also on the parish board at the Indian Hill Church and a co-chair of the Altar Guild.

She was preceded in death by her husband, Charles G. Puchta, in 1997. In addition to her son, survivors include: a daughter, Polly Puchta Wells of Loveland and six grandchildren. A memorial service is 10:30 a.m. Wednesday at the Indian Hill Episcopal-Presbyterian Church, 6000 Drake Road. Interment will be at Walnut Hills Cemetery. Memorials: Alois Alzheimer's Center, 70 Damon Road, Cincinnati 45218.

It's Never too Late

A friend of mine once made the statement that it is never too late to be the person you might have been. This is often times true of people who take the time and effort to prepare their own obituary in advance of their death. One famous story is the story of Alfred Noble. According the website www.enchantedspirit.org, *"An interesting moment of personal examination came to Alfred Nobel one morning when we woke to find his own obituary reported in a French newspaper. "Alfred Noble, the inventor of dynamite, who died yesterday, devised a way for more people to be killed in a war than ever before, and he died a very rich man.""* What happened was the newspaper mistakenly reported the death of Alfred when in fact his brother Ludvig Noble actually died. The story goes on the *"As Noble's health deteriorated, his guilt over what looked to be the final legacy of his life escalated. A little over a year before he died, Alfred Nobel drew up....the Will establishing what would become the Noble Prize...a series of awards for individuals whose contributions inspire the world." "Every man ought to have the chance, he said, to correct his epitaph in midstream and write a new one."* So the question is if you write your obituary today, would you want it to say something different? If you answered yes, there may still be time to be the person you might have been.

Big Picture Considerations

To prepare for the death of a loved one, give consideration to the needs of the surviving spouse. Providing for a surviving spouse can be a primary responsibility that is overlooked. Life insurance is one tool to help ensure survivors have the necessary financial resources to carry on. Ensure beneficiary designations are up-to-date and on file. In addition to financial responsibilities, give consideration to the type of daily activities that a loved one may not have much experience. For example, when my father died, my mother would not have been comfortable handling the daily finances and any type of legal or insurance decisions. Likewise, if my mother had predeceased my dad, he would not have been comfortable handling the grocery shopping, cooking, laundry and day-to-day household responsibilities.

Summary

End-of-life should not be a lonely, painful or traumatic experience for people and their families. I believe that families should always strive to ensure a person is comfortable and maintains his or her dignity and respect. Consider the many advantages of Hospice Care and decide if it may be appropriate for your family.

Even though death is inevitable, death is a subject that most people would rather not discuss. One reason may be the fear of the unknown. For others, they fear that acknowledging and discussing death may in essence be suggesting a readiness as if death with occur sooner rather than later. Death is the great equalizer. No longer does one's career, education, accumulations make a difference. The only thing that is sustaining is our relationships. Take the time to consider pre-planning a funeral and give consideration to the many options in advance. Consider how a person will be remembered and write an obituary and eulogy in advance of a loved one's death.

When a loved one dies, you will find that there is a lot to do and a short period of time to do it in. I encourage you to give advance consideration to planning a funeral. Don't let a death be more overwhelming more than it already is.

> *When my father passed away I quickly came to realize everything that had to be done to make a tribute to his life. As such, I found that I had no time to mourn his death as I was too busy running all over town gathering information for his obituary, preparing my remarks for the memorial service and making arrangements for the funeral, family luncheon that followed, etc. Once the memorial service was over, three days later, I literally fell on my face I was so exhausted and emotionally drained.*

KEY LEARNINGS – *Top three learnings from this chapter:*
1.
2.
3.

ACTION ITEMS - *Things you want to do, or do differently:*		
Check when Completed	*Action Item*	*Target Completion Date*

11

The Talk

Open and honest communication between family members is critically important. Many people simply don't seem to understand that for their wishes to be carried out; they need to share their wishes. If you are, or anticipate being, a caregiver and your loved one has not shared his wishes, maybe it's time for you to start asking a few questions. Family is usually the most affected by the important decisions and is called upon at some point to provide help.

While family discussions can often be challenging and uncomfortable, having 'the talk' enables family members to understand a loved one's wishes and gain points of view that may not have been considered. If your family is not much on discussing personal matters and you have concern about interfering with a loved one's personal matter, ask yourself a simple question; *"how are you going to know what your loved one would want and how to help?"*

While I entitle this chapter 'The Talk,' maybe I should have called it 'The Talks,' suggesting the plural, not singular. Having an initial conversation or family meeting is a great start, but you are likely to have many talks over the course of time. While there may be lots of things you'd like to know and discuss, be careful not to overwhelm a loved one. It might be helpful to think about the talk as peeling back the layers of an onion. Think about the few key questions you might have as you get started. Then as you have the opportunity to go deeper in the future, you can delve into other questions and concerns.

Many parents do not want to talk about aging and long-term care as it may represent a fear of losing independence or being an invasion of privacy. I equate the talk Baby Boomers need to have with their parents with the talk that our parents had with us years ago about the Birds and the Bees. I think the analogy of the two 'talks' is quite relevant for a couple of reasons.

1. The talk is not intended to be easy and spur of the moment. It is something that people should plan for, take seriously and realize that loved ones may soon enter a new stage in life, if they haven't already.

2. The first few words can make it or break it. Either you get someone's attention and there is a mutual appreciation for having a conversation, or the barriers go up and not much will be accomplished.

The point of the talk is ultimately to understand a loved one's wishes and expectations. Everything else should be secondary. Unfortunately many conversations are derailed as the talk becomes focused on money and inheritance. Be careful. Recognize that when the topic of money comes up, some parents may feel their kids are selfish in their motives.

If the discussion goes off on tangents, or becomes uncomfortable or hostile, you might suggest a few reasons for wanting to have the conversation, such as:

- To ensure a loved one has completed some sort of estate planning and legal planning.

- To understand and be able to carry out a loved one's health care wishes should he become incapable of making his own decisions.

Basic Questions to Ask

Basic things you will want to determine during conversations include:

1. If something ever happens to you, what would you want me (or us, as a family) to do? What are the roles and expectations you have for family members in terms of providing assistance, support, and the like?

2. Have you executed legal documents including a Will, Power of Attorney, Living Will and Power of Attorney for Health Care?

    a. If YES, where are copies of the documents located? Where is the original Will located? Who is appointed to make decisions for you should you be unable?

    b.   If NO, encourage your parent or loved on to execute the basic documents (See Chapter #7)

3.   Have you planned for long-term care? What are your wishes should you become less independent and require some sort of care? Do you have a preference in terms of living environment and/or care option(s)? What type of arrangements are the least desirable?

4.   Are there any medical conditions that you are currently facing or predisposed to from your family that might be an indicator of future challenges?

5.   Have you planned for your retirement and saved money to cover your typical expenses? Do you have a budget? What type of assumptions have you factored in your retirement plan in regards to living and care expenses? (e.g., how many years you assumed your money will need to last – projected life expectancy? What are your expectations for personal expenses)

6.   What types of assets are at your disposal should you need funds to cover any sort of care expenses? (e.g., cash value in life insurance, long-term care insurance, equity in a house)

7.   What type of health insurance do you have and do you expect it to be sufficient for the future?

8.   If anything happens to you, what would your wishes be for mom/dad? Are there concerns you have that you would like the family to be aware of?

These are some fundamental questions that, at a minimum, every family should discuss. I intentionally suggest the questions be somewhat general for the first talk. If a loved one has not given much consideration to the questions and issues, you might share this Resource Guide, and encourage your parent to consider the questions above. Also, if one parent names the other parent in their legal documents, it might be wise to name a back-up person just in case. If parents have divorced and remarried, make sure the wishes are clear in terms of both children and step children.

Who Should Participate?

One of the first things you and your family should determine is who should participate in family meetings? There are no right or wrong answers. Depending on the intended topic of conversation, certain people may or may not be included. So what are some options to consider?

- Talks may take place between family members that do not include the current or potential care recipient. For example, adult children might get together to discuss when to have the initial conversation, who might be most appropriate to initiate the idea of having a talk, and what to cover in an initial discussion.

- Certain topics of conversation such as financial matters may be limited to the immediate family.

- Conversations having to do with a loved one's day-to-day care might include the parents, children, in-laws, step children, friends, neighbors and anyone else who could be a potential caregiver, regardless of how large or small their role.

- If certain family members live out of town, you might need to make decisions about moving forward with or without a particular relative.

Regardless of who is involved in conversations, plan an agenda and share it in advance of your discussion to give participants time to plan and prepare. Remember, you don't want to ambush anyone. An agenda might include the following topics and flow:

1. Current Situation - What is the latest on a person's medical diagnosis and prognosis? Are there certain changes or events which merit discussion or review?

2. Feelings Check – How is everyone feeling? (e.g., overwhelmed, scared, sad, etc.)

3. Needs – What needs to be done or done differently? Why? Does everyone agree? What is the goal or desired outcome from the conversation? Are there certain financial or legal concerns that need to be addressed? Is one person asking for responsibility to be shared by others?

4. Roles and Responsibilities – Who wants to do what? What specific limitations do people have in regards to time or location that need to be recognized? Who is going to do what in terms of making decisions, coordinating care, handling personal affairs, interacting with the medical team? Also, how often is each family member planning to contact a parent by telephone or in person?

5. Agreement – divide and conquer. Agree how to keep everyone up-to-date. Plan the next meeting.

The Talk

Don't try to do too much at any one meeting. I like to refer to a meeting as a conversation or talk as opposed to a meeting simply due to formality associated with the term meeting. Remember you are dealing with real people. Maintain structure and purpose but be careful not to come across as rigid and impersonal.

Make sure everyone has a chance to be heard. If a particular family member is more outspoken, maybe another family member needs to ask him or her to give other people a chance to be heard. Consider the "here and now" and the future. Don't waste time looking back and pointing blame. An agenda is important because to helps to focus the conversation.

Depending on the topic and participants, the purpose of an initial conversation might simply be to gain consensus that there is a need to talk on an on-going basis and that there are potentially real issues that the family will want to address.

Have Reasonable Expectations

While family discussion can be an effective and essential way to get family members together, don't expect miracles to happen. Use the tools provided throughout this Resource Guide in addition to turning to professionals for assistance.

> *I was fortunate in that my dad initiated the talk about personal and financial affairs. While he provided copies of both his and mom's Wills and other advance directives, I never thought to ask more questions about his wishes regarding health care and end-of-life. When he passed away I discovered a number of things I had not known such as he recently purchased a long-term care insurance policy for my mom. Also, he had never shared with us that his family had long ago purchased cemetery plots.*

An article entitled <u>Oh, grow up!</u> by Sarah Sabalos of the Knight Rider News Service offered advice to adult children desiring a healthy, peer relationship with their parents.

- *"Avoid topics and conversations you know are problematic*
- *Decide what's worth arguing about and what you should ignore*
- *Acknowledge what your mother says, but don't overreact.*
- *Weight how much of the annoyance comes from your mother and how much is actually pressure you are putting on yourself.*

- *Bear in mind, it's not important that you always be "right."*
- *Don't be afraid to ruffle your mother's feathers*
- *Be aware of what you want from your mother and what she is capable and prepared to give."*

Communication Guidelines

Talking about one's personal affairs can be awkward for many families. The outcome of a conversation shouldn't be 'my way,' 'no way,' 'half way,' or 'your way.' It seems that participants are often focused on 'winning' or 'losing' as opposed to understanding each others points of view and perspectives, and reaching agreement.

I encourage families to follow the Respectful Communication Guidelines that were developed by the Rev. Eric H.F. Law an Episcopal priest and author.

R – Take responsibility for what you say and feel without blaming others

  (Use "I" statements, not "you")

E – Empathetic listening.

S – Be sensitive to differences in communication styles

P – Ponder what you hear and feel before you speak

E – Examine your own assumptions and perceptions

  (Why am I reacting/feeling this way?)

C – Keep confidentiality to uphold the wellbeing of the community

T – Tolerate ambiguity because we are not here to debate who is right or wrong.

Caregiver Considerations

Because only one of ten people dies suddenly, ninety percent of us can expect to face health care decisions as we approach the end of our lives. Take time to understand a loved one's wishes and desires for long-term care. When talking with family, consider your tone when speaking. Use "I" statements instead of "You" statements and avoid misinterpretation by being simple, clear and concise. Build cooperation by addressing issues where there is likely to be agreement. Then, as momentum builds, discuss more challenging or controversial issues.

The Talk

Caregivers should give consideration to their schedules and ability to provide the necessary care. A question I encourage caregivers to ask themselves is, given my responsibilities, commitments and time constraints, how much help can I reasonably give? How much am I willing to give?

In addition to yourself and your siblings, ask other family members and friends if they are willing and able to help. Consider how much help and support the care recipient is willing to accept.

If you are a caregiver, remember that the care recipient has the right and responsibility to make all decisions, as long as he or she has the mental capacity to do so.

Engaging A Loved One

After establishing the agenda, decide how to engage a loved in a conversation or family meeting. I find that the way family members engage, or attempt to engage each other, can be as important to consider as the discussion itself. The following three approaches tend to work well. Determine which, if any of these approaches, may work best for you.

1. SCRIPTED – With the scripted approach, you plan ahead and give advance notification to your loved ones that you would like to talk or have a family meeting. I believe that advance notice is critical so no one feels ambushed, caught off guard, unprepared or backed into a corner. With this approach, you simply call a loved one and request a get together to talk. For people that attend my seminars, I suggest that they say something like: *"Hey Dad, I was at a seminar last week on the topic of long-term care and I got to thinking that there are a lot of things I don't know that I probably should know. Can we get together over the weekend and talk? I'd like to ask you some questions and find out your preferences and expectations should anything ever happen to you or mom."* With this approach, both parties have a chance to reflect and prepare. When you arrive for the talk, there should be no surprise when you start asking questions.

2. SPONTANEOUS – Many people seem to have their guard up and may not be interested in sharing or discussing personal matters. When this occurs, look for a situation that hits close to home emotionally that might impact your loved one. For my dad, the situation was the death of one of his best friends. When my dad learned of his friend's death, many realities appeared to have set in, enabling me to see the softer side

of dad. This was my opportunity to come along side my dad, and tell him that as a result of his friends death, *"I now realize that there are many things I don't know about your and mom's wishes should anything ever happen to either of you."* Then, immediately start asking questions or agree to sit down in a week or so to talk.

3. LEAD BY EXAMPLE – Get your own personal affairs in order so you are able to speak from experience. In this case, you might be able to share some of your plans and documents. For example, I could have said to my dad, *"I have planned and organized my personal affairs for the benefit of Karen (my wife) and our daughters should anything ever happen to me. Can I talk to you about some of the things I have done to make life easier should I predecease Karen? Also, I would like to talk to you about your wishes should you predecease mom?"* If you are unsure what, if anything, your loved one has planned or considered, you may ask, *"have you given much consideration to your wishes and what you would like or expect me to do?"*

Consider where to hold a discussion so that everyone is comfortable and in an appropriate setting. A private setting such as a home or office may provide less distractions, whereas a public setting or neutral site, avoid any 'home field' advantage.

If a person seems reluctant to talk about himself, it may be easier to talk about the spouse. Ask dad about mom, what his wishes for her might be should anything happen to him. Removing dad as the topic of conversation, and focusing on mom, can often be an effective way to get a conversation started.

Regardless of the approach or setting, during the talk with your parent, try not to come across as threatening, controlling, selfish, or condescending. Coming across inappropriately or forcefully can derail a conversation before it even gets started.

Families Are Different
What may work best for one family could flop for another. Each family has a unique history and dynamic that affects family interactions. Different people respond differently to conversations about care and end-of-life issues. If your family is having a hard time reaching agreement, I suggest you consider using the Decision Spectrum tool presented in Chapter #2.

If you come from what might be considered a dysfunctional family, don't be surprised if the conversation is challenging. If you tend to talk more about news, weather and sports when engaging with family, it may be awkward talking about real concerns that have the potential to impact a person's life. It is amazing how things that were done years and years ago can lead to resentment or favoritism. While conflict may make difficult decisions even harder, I still suggest family members work through issues, rather than ignore them.

If family personalities may impede a productive conversation, consider engaging the services of a Geriatric Care Manager or a Social Worker. Unbiased outsiders may be able to help facilitate discussions and provide counsel to your family.

Convincing A Loved One to Accept Help

An older person's reluctance to accept help creates conflict for the adult children who are attempting to provide support. However, concerns about a person's health, safety and well-being make it appropriate and even necessary to bring up topics that older adults would rather not discuss. A good starting place is to talk about your own feelings, concerns and needs. For example: *"Mom, I am worried about your going up and down the stairs because you might fall and hurt yourself. With your osteoporosis you could get badly hurt. I'd like to talk with you about hiring someone to do the laundry for you, so you don't have to go down to the basement."* At the same time, bring up fears which may not have been expressed, such as *"This doesn't mean I want you to move to a nursing home. I want to help you stay in your home."* Getting the issues out on the table gives families a chance to discuss issues, even though it may be uncomfortable at first. Even though it may be simple for you to see a workable solution for someone else, your point of view might not take into consideration the things your loved one is thinking and experiencing.

Encourage family members to talk and be willing to explore ways to accommodate a loved one's wishes whenever possible and realistic. Encourage care recipients to participate in arranging for services that are needed so they feel involved. It is important for everyone to feel that we are in control of our own lives. The worst thing caregivers can do is try to force someone to do something against their will. Power struggles rarely, if ever, work. Try to be understanding and optimistic at all times. Address a loved one's objections or hesitations creatively, rather than arguing with them.

Parent's Refusal

I constantly hear from people indicating that a parent refuses to do something such as see a doctor or make a change in life to get out of a bad situation. People often get frustrated that a loved one refuses to do something that may seem so obvious. So what do you do when that happens?

- Don't try to do anything behind someone's back (e.g., hire a caregiver, try to purchase long-term care (LTC) insurance.) Instead, have a heart to heart talk with them, and encourage them to do something different.

- Don't try to tell them what 'they need to do' or come across suggesting that they do what you're telling them. Instead, try making a plea for them to do something for YOU, not for themselves.

In other words, indicate that without LTC insurance, if anything happens to them, the burden/responsibility will be on you to provide for their care. It is as though you are asking them for a favor – please do this for me. If they still flat out refuse your suggestions consider modifying something that you do for them. In other words, if you won't have the courtesy to let me purchase LTC insurance for you, them I won't be able to *(...insert something that they value...)* for you. People often cut off contact with grandkids, reduce the frequency of visits, etc. so that the parent can't have their cake and eat it too.

A lot of times the things an older parent or loved one does may be out of fear. For example if they are appearing selfish, maybe they fear losing your companionship. If you are feeling under the control or influence of an older adult that makes you feel like a child, maybe it's time to put your foot down and stop taking orders and reacting to each and every whim. Set ground rules and establish boundaries. Know your limits and make sure you don't sacrifice your own life. Also, be aware of the alternatives. Often times, the care receiver has everything to lose and nothing to gain, however, they are the ones making the demands.

Summary

It is often difficult for people to talk about long-term care as it represents a fear of loss of independence. As a result, do not be surprised if your parents are reluctant to want to talk with you about the future. For men especially, talking about care can appear to be a sign of weakness whereby they allow themselves to become vulnerable.

Give consideration to who should participate in discussions and what you want to accomplish as a result of a talk. Whenever you talk to a parent about his or her personal affairs, be careful not to come across as threatening, controlling, selfish, or condescending. Some experts suggest that adult children get their own affairs in order first so that they are able to speak from experience. Once you have your personal affairs in order, you might offer to show him what you have done to make life easier for your family should you predecease your spouse, and ask for the same courtesy in return.

While the topic of money will eventually emerge, I suggest focusing initial discussions on understanding a parent's long-term care wishes so you are in a position to honor his or her wishes. When the topic of money does occur, as it eventually should, encourage your loved ones to clearly document their wishes so that there assets and personal property are handling according to their wishes. Ideally you should convey that you are more interested in making sure they are cared for and their wishes are fulfilled than receiving a share of their assets.

Misunderstanding or miscommunication can be devastating to family relationships. Also, sibling rivalry that could date back years and years could come up. For example, one sibling may harbor resentment and have an attitude like Mom always liked you best anyway. If trying to express yourself and get beyond what ever has kept you apart, speak frankly – say what you mean, mean what you say, just don't be mean when you say it. Also, don't come across as though you have all the answers. Remember people have two ears and only one mouth. Ask questions and be open to another's thoughts and ideas. Ask – What's your take on this whole thing? What do you suggest?

KEY LEARNINGS – *Top three learnings from this chapter:*

1.	
2.	
3.	

ACTION ITEMS - *Things you want to do, or do differently:*

Check when Completed	Action Item	Target Completion Date

#12

Emotional Challenges

People tend to discount many of the emotional challenges both care recipients and caregivers face. Many people refer to caregiving as a journey, suggesting that people will face a variety of challenges over time and that you never know quite what to expect. People also associate caregiving with a roller coaster ride as there are twists, turns, and ups and downs. My hope is that this Resource Guide provides you with new information, and encourages you to take whatever steps are most appropriate for your situation. Hopefully, you are gaining an awareness and understanding of the many options, considerations and decision points, so you are in a better position to make informed decisions either with or for a loved one.

First, do not try to figure everything out by yourself. Reach out to others. Do not to isolate yourself and handle everything independently. Remember, everyone who takes on the role of family caregiver is inexperienced. Just as the Lone Ranger didn't go though life alone, he had Tonto, make sure you have a side kick or two.

Webster's definition of emotion is *"A mental state that arises spontaneously rather than through conscious effort, and is often accompanied by physiological changes; a feeling: the emotion of joy, sorrow, reverence, hate and love."*

I begin with the definition to highlight the spontaneity of emotions. Emotions can not be controlled, just they just happen. Still, take time to acknowledge your emotions and work through them. Do not overlook your emotions and let them percolate inside of you. Also, don't get angry toward someone who is impaired or otherwise faces limitations; after all, it's not their fault.

Care Recipient Perspectives

I strongly encourage care recipients and caregivers alike to watch the movie <u>On Golden Pond</u>. Even though you may have watched it years ago, watch it again to observe and appreciate the challenges an older person may face. Henry Fonda, portraying the role of Mr. Thayer, is simply spectacular. There is the scene where he is walking in the woods and gets confused and lost. There is another scene where Sumner, the kid at the General Store and Gas Dock insults Mr. Thayer. These scenes and many more throughout the movie are priceless. In the gas dock scene, Mr. Thayer makes a comment in regards to the high price of gas. He says *"Do you know what gas cost when I was your age? $0.12 cents a gallon."* Sumner responds by saying *"I didn't know they had gas back then."* Then Mr. Thayer makes a priceless comment. *"Do you think it is funny being old? My whole gosh darn body is falling apart. Heck I can't even go to the bathroom when I want to. But I'm still a man and I can take you on."*

The reason why I mention this scene is to again, reinforce perspectives and emotions of the care recipients. If people, primarily caregivers, had a different perspective, they might do things differently keeping in contact with and supporting a care recipient.

The common emotion of fear manifests itself in many ways.
- As a response to learning of a medical diagnosis and the associated uncertainty of life, concern about pain, etc.
- As a response to being forgotten.
- As a response to being left alone, especially upon the death of a spouse.
- As a response to the uncertainty associated with death.

Frustration is another common emotion.
- Frustration experiencing physical or psychological limitations.
- Frustration with dependency on others. For example, waiting on results from medical tests or waiting in a medical office to see the doctor.
- Frustration when a spouse or child wants or suggests something that is inconsistent with what a care recipient wishes.

Be aware of the many emotions a care recipient may encounter over time. Also, recognize that if a loved one experiences an emotion, it is real to him, regardless if it is real to you.

Caregiver Guilt

A common caregiver emotion is guilt. Quite often guilt is associated with things people don't do, as much as it is associated with things people actually do. For example, a family member may feel guilty if he or she doesn't make the time to visit with Mom and Dad on a regular basis. Reasons why people may not want to go visit Mom may include the following:

- You always feel guilty when its time to go.

- It is depressing to see your loved one in her condition.

- You feel guilty that maybe Mom should be living somewhere else or be receiving different care, but that may not be feasible financially.

- Maybe the relationship is broken and it is time for reconciliation.

- Maybe starting and keeping a conversation is difficult.

Caregivers may also feel guilty when taking time and attention for themselves, or acting against the expressed wishes of a loved one because you believe in your heart, what you are doing is in her best interest. Sometimes, caregivers even blame themselves for the loved one's illness. Caregivers should try to keep things in perspective such as:

- Realize that you are just one person and can only do so much.

- Spend time preparing yourself and consider the predominant issues and challenges you are likely to face, to avoid or minimize crisis situations.

- Do not be afraid to frequently ask for help.

- Recognize all your responsibilities (e.g. spouse, kids, work,), not just being a family caregiver, and schedule your time.

- Set reasonable expectations for yourself to minimize your frustration.

- Realize that you are not perfect, and give yourself permission to make mistakes.

- Recognize your many accomplishments and take pride in the rewards of caring for a loved one.

As I said earlier, be aware of your guilty feelings as much as possible. Otherwise, they may build up inside, causing you to feel resentful, angry and frustrated. Negative feelings can interfere with a caregiver's ability and desire to provide nurturing care, and may result in misplaced hostility toward the loved one he or she is trying to help.

Caregiver Perspectives

Caregivers are often conflicted if, or when, a loved one is not accepting of the help and suggestions being offered. People have been taught to *"Honor Your Mother and Father,"* *"Obey Your Parents"* and *"Respect Your Elders"* from the time they are children. Then a loved one says *"I'm fine"* when he clearly isn't fine. The question then becomes, what do I do? I believe that honoring, obeying and respecting a loved one may not simply be to roll over and accept whatever the care recipient requests. I believe adult children have a responsibility to look out for their parent's best interests, whether it is doing what is popular or unpopular.

Remember that as long as the care recipient is of clear mind and deemed competent, he or she ultimately has final say, whether you as a caregiver like it and agree with a loved one's choices or not. I believe the best way to approach any decisions is by following the Golden Rule. *"Do unto other's as you would have them do unto you."* While it is clearly subjective in terms of what is in someone's best interest, the best test can often be looking into the mirror and asking yourself if what you are doing or suggesting is consistent to how you would want someone to treat you in the same situation.

Caregivers face a number of emotions. In Chapter #3 I brought attention to the difference between the words 'Need' and 'Want.' Here again, I suggest you recognize the words you use when you talk. A common scenario I witness is when a person says *"I need to go visit Mom this weekend."* When I hear that, I typically respond by saying *"Stop, don't go."* The point is that if you are going because you perceive your reason for going to be a need, you might want to reconsider. When someone uses the word 'Need,' a person making the visit seems to be set that he is going to make a 20 minute visit and the clock starts counting when the car enters the driveway. What I instead suggest, is changing the statement and instead saying *"I Want to go visit Mom today."* If substituting the word 'Want' for 'Need' makes the statement false, it may be worth figuring out why deep down inside, you don't want to go.

Maybe something happened or something was said during a visit that led you to feel a certain way that makes you feel uncomfortable, or brings back an old and painful memory. I am always amazed how a parent or spouse can say a few simple words that can get under a person's skin in a matter of seconds. Everything may be going along fine then, wham, out of nowhere, an emotional nerve is hit. For example, it is not uncommon for someone to say something like *"Don't worry about me"* which may mean the exact opposite and invoke an emotion of guilt.

Caregivers also have some wonderfully positive emotions as well. A common, positive emotion caregivers feel is joy. Joy from being able to provide care and assistance to someone who gave much of her life, time and treasure, to raise you. Often times, when a crisis occurs, it causes people to stop and look at life. Are your priorities in order? Are you using your time wisely? Crisis situations often bring a family together and get family members to look past the things that have happened, and look ahead to the future and how to make the most of each new day.

Boundaries

Many people I speak with indicate they feel guilty about their emotions, or that their emotions are making them not like themselves. As you consider your emotions, it is important to understand and identify any underlying circumstance causing the emotion. For example, a friend's mother-in-law is living with him and his wife. While she has her own apartment in the basement, she feels it necessary to tell him and his wife how to parent their children. Also, she will call upstairs on numerous occasions each day, to ask questions and speak with her daughter. He realizes that he and his wife need to establish healthy boundaries with the mother-in-law, and not let her comments and calls get to them. In this situation, my friend has validated his feelings, worked through his feelings, and has established a solution to help him get past his feelings. For more on boundaries, I recommend the book entitled <u>Boundaries</u> by Dr. Henry Cloud.

One saying that I love is: *"Say what you mean. Mean what you say. Just don't say it mean."* Whatever the circumstance, if you can understand what the underlying fear or frustration might be, you can start to address it. Don't hesitate to talk about what's going on.

Mental Health

Let me share a quick story that might help put some of the emotional or mental challenges into perspective. When my wife and I had young children, we got together with four other couples on a weekly basis. During our time together, we each shared what is going in our lives, including those things that were challenging us, and the things that had brought us great joy. Since everyone in the group had young children, we were always so relieved to learn that other people's kids act up, do not understand the word 'NO,' or are unwilling to sit still for a meal, etc. What happens is 'Validation' - the, *"I'm okay, you're okay process".* Regardless of whether the issues are small kids or aging parents, validation can be so critical when you are faced with challenges.

Do not overlook your mental health, or the mental health of the care recipient. The following is a story from the January 3, 2003 edition of The Cincinnati Enquirer.

Man, wife leap to their deaths from Fla. Condo.

Hollywood FL., On the last day of 2002, 85-year-old xxx had a maintenance worker open the windows and remove the screens in his 17th-floor condominium. Mr. xxx, who had lung disease, explained that he needed more fresh air. Then, three hours before the new year, Mr. xxx leaped to his death, followed seconds later by his 80-year-old wife, Estelle. The couple of 42 years had been in failing health, and Mr. xxx was becoming increasingly feeble. The two left a note with burial instructions.

I don't like reading this kind of story; however, it points out and reminds us of the realities many people are facing. In fact, suicide is a very real issue for Senior Citizens. According to the National Institute of Mental Health, approximately 20% of all suicides in the US are committed by individuals aged 65 and older. Older men are almost four times more likely than women to die by suicide. *"At higher risk are elders who live alone, have suffered a major interpersonal loss, lack a supportive social system and/or are facing a terminal decline."* Source: Kastenbaum, Robert, <u>Dying and Bereavement,</u> Gerontology: An Interdisciplinary Perspective, New York: Oxford Press.

Coping & Helping

Coping can be especially difficult for families dealing with a chronic illness. Mrs. Audrey Kron, a Detroit area medical psychotherapist and author of a book entitled <u>Meeting the Challenge: Living with Chronic Illness</u> (www.ChronicIllness.com) suggests a few coping mechanisms:

- Try to live your live as normally as you can

- Be prepared

- Pour your feelings into a creative outlet

Don't think solely about your loved one; also consider yourself and your needs and feelings. An unhealthy caregiver is of no value to a care recipient. Caregiving is sure to take an emotional toll on you. To help validate yourself, and recognize that you're not alone, I recommend participating in a support group, at least once in a while. Also, there are programs like respite care (discussed in the previous chapter) which can be extremely valuable to caregivers.

An example that is often used to demonstrate the importance of the caregiver taking care of herself is from the airline industry. When the flight attendant is explaining the safety procedures, he or she says *"in the event a cabin depressurization, air masks will automatically fall from above. If this happens, place your own mask securely around your head before tending to those around you."* The point is that caregivers must make their own health and well-being a priority.

Don't beat yourself up if the care needed is beyond what you can provide. You will likely wonder if anyone can provide the same loving care as you. After all, you have years and years of experience with your parent, now along comes someone that doesn't know her, her feelings, likes, dislikes, etc.

Another emotion many caregivers face is when a parent is forced to make a move because of a medical condition. For example, we moved my mom to a Retirement Community which had a unit that specialized in dementia care. My sister and I had quite a difficult time dealing with the fact that mom would now be living in a 400 square foot room in a rather sterile environment. Our challenge was that our mom deserved better or more. Having lived in a nice middle class home all her life, we found it tremendously difficult to see her having to leave the majority of her possessions behind. Basically, she was able to have a bed, chair, table, and a few pictures.

Outside Support

Don't internalize everything and let things get bottled up inside of you. Identify resources and support groups in your area. You'll quickly find that most people are ready and eager to help you. To locate support groups in your area, ask a local senior agency or refer to the Health and Wellness section featured weekly in many local newspapers. Also, seek morale support from family and friends. Talk about the emotions you are experiencing, and get things off your chest when you feel burdened.

Big Picture Considerations

Caregivers can expect to experience a variety of emotions along their journey. I vividly remember when my sister and I moved our mom into a dementia care unit at a local nursing home. Once the move was complete, our mom looked at us and said *"please don't leave."* Wow, talk about an emotional challenge when I walked out the door. Another comment my mom would make was *"You're coming back tomorrow, right?"* When comments like that were made, I often felt guilty if I wasn't planning on visiting the following day. Another struggle I faced was how to respond. I never wanted to lie, but at the same time, I didn't want mom to be lonely or be away from people who loved her.

If a parent has limited financial resources, adult children can often struggle to determine how much they can and should provide in terms of financial assistance. It can be emotionally challenging for a child to live a comfortable middle class life, and realize that mom or dad is just barely able to make ends meet. That is why in Chapter #11, I indicate the importance of having the talk and developing an awareness of a parent's personal and financial affairs. In terms of assistance, whether financial or otherwise, I can only recommend to apply the Golden Rule: Do unto others as you would have them do unto you.

An unexpected emotion is the feeling some people experience when they receive an inheritance. If you are likely to receive an inheritance, prepare emotionally and financially. In addition to grieving over the loss of a loved one, many people experience guilt from gaining materially from it. Some experience anger and view it as unfair that mom and dad didn't do more for themselves. Many couples that receive inheritance have conflict when it comes time to deciding if they are going to save or spend the inheritance.

Also, when a loved one dies, it is important for family members to grieve their loss, and not simply stuff their feelings. I talk about grief in detail in Chapter #14 entitled Facing Death.

Summary

Caregivers often get so wrapped up in providing care that they experience feelings of isolation, loneliness, depression and more. Support group meetings provide a fabulous forum to help you deal with your issues and feelings.

Prepare yourself for a bumpy ride. You are sure to face unexpected challenges along your journey. That is a normal part of caregiving. If you get frustrated with a situation and have any anger or animosity against your loved one, ask yourself a simple question: Do you really think that your parents want to be a burden on you? Few people answer yes. As such, you may simply need to realize that as people face mental or physical challenges, many simply cannot cope.

Recognize that you may need to make some tough and unpopular decisions. I recommend being gentle, kind and compassionate in all that you do. The following is an excerpt from a card I received years ago that indicates just how crazy things can get:

"Regarding Granny…we have moved her into her new "home at SunRise. Of course we had to trick her to get her there & secretly bring all of her personal things, which was a heart wrenching episode due to all of our emotions. Lots of tears that day, but I'm happy to report that none have been shed since. (At least none regarding her living arrangement.) Unbelievably, she is rather happy…very content. Thank God for that! As you know (unfortunately) Alzheimer's is an extremely sad and painful thing to watch your loved one go through. But, with God's Grace, we have all learned to love, accept, embrace and cherish our "new" Granny."

KEY LEARNINGS – *Top three learnings from this chapter:*

1.
2.
3.

ACTION ITEMS - *Things you want to do, or do differently:*

Check when Completed	Action Item	Target Completion Date

13

Legacy of Memories

Think about your parent's life, and you can quickly find yourself immersed on a sentimental journey. With the hustle and bustle of life, many people do not spend adequate time capturing memories. Then something happens and it's too late. I have a simple recommendation. Think about things you might do, starting today, to make the most of each and every day.

If I have heard it once, I have heard it a thousand times. Someone is hospitalized or is diagnosed with an illness, and all of a sudden the entire family is re-evaluating and re-prioritizing everything in life. People start to make time for things that have previously been overlooked, or not given an appropriate amount of attention. When a crisis occurs, the reality of life and death often sets in and people come to realize what is important in life.

How can you make the most of each new day? Do you find your conversation centers around news, weather and sports, as opposed to life? Are there certain memories that you would like to preserve forever? A wonderful book I suggest is <u>Tuesdays with Morrie</u> written by Mitch Albom. I found this book to be a life changing book about life's simple lessons. The book is about a gentleman, a professor, who had ALS (Lou Gehrig's disease) and how he and a former student would get together on Tuesdays during the last year of the professor's life to talk about life. The topic of discussion for each get together was determined in advance, and the conversations and learnings were fascinating each week. So much wisdom, it's incredible.

What is sad is that many people simply never take the time to tap into the wisdom and life experiences of loved ones. Spending time with your loved one reminiscing about the past can be a most rewarding experience.

- Imagine what life must have been like before television, VCR's, Velcro, microwave ovens, computers, fast food? Oh how the world has changed!

- Imagine what it would have been like having your milk and eggs delivered fresh to your doorstep.

- Imagine what it must have been like going on vacation and not having the luxury of having a TV and VCR in the car to entertain the kids?

- Imagine what it must have been like living during the Great Depression and the years that followed?

People that have served in the Armed Forces also have lived through incredible experiences that helped shape our world and protect our freedom. Many people take for granted certain memories or stories that they have heard a hundred times before. However, once it comes time to repeat the story, you have trouble with the specific details. Or, people may take for granted that a parent knows how you feel, how grateful you are for the life your parents made possible.

As people have come to realize, especially since the September 11th tragedy, we cannot take anyone's life for granted. Tomorrow is not a sure thing. With that in mind, are there things you want to say? Questions you want to ask? Things you would like to do?

Simple Things To Do

Death can be uncertain in that people never know when, how, or where it will strike. To families with aging parents, I suggest a few things. At your next family gathering, whether it is a birthday, holiday or other occasion, consider the following:

- Pull out a camera and take a few extra pictures.

- Talk from your heart, and let your parent know how you feel.

- Ask a few questions to help you remember stories accurately and in colorful detail.

Legacy of Memories

The following is a Dear Abby column from June 20, 2002:

Dear Abby: During my mother's fight with breast cancer, she was in and out of hospitals. My sister made a 3-by-4 foot collage of old photographs of family, friends and places that Mom loved to visit. This collage went with her from hospital room to hospital room for the duration of her illness.

It served to remind everyone that Mom was once a vibrant lady with a rich, full life, who was loved by all the people pictured. She was cheered up by it and it served to "humanize' her to the myriad of doctors, nurses, aides and technicians who treated her.

Now that Mom is gone, the collage is hung in a prominent place in our family home. It serves as a constant reminder of how much we love and miss her.

-   Dave in Ohio.

Dear Dave: I'm sure your sister's masterpiece is a treasure, and will continue to be considered so by future generations.

Pull Out A Camera

Once our father passed away, my sister realized that she never had a picture of Gramps and her youngest daughter, even though she had a picture of Gramps alone with her other two children. Unfortunately it was too late. They had video of certain events, but not others, but again, it was too late. Photographs and video are memories you can cherish forever. Therefore, do not wait until a loved one has passed before you realize you have not captured certain memories on film. Take a minute now to think which pictures you might cherish that you do not already have.

At your next gathering, pull out a video camera and turn it on. You do not need to tell your mom and dad that you are capturing memories to enjoy once they have passed away. Rather, use it as an opportunity to ask you parent's questions about their life, childhood, how they met, and more. Ask about how you were as a child, what they remember most, your first words, and other fond memories. You will be glad you did. It is always nice to be able to hear someone's voice long after they are gone.

Talk from your Heart

Once a loved one has passed, it will be too late to tell him how much you love him, appreciate him and all the things he has done for you throughout your life. All too often in this fast paced world, people take things for granted. Many families have assumed all their lives that they love each other, even though it is rarely spoken.

Make sure you say what is in your heart before it is too late. *"I Love You"* are powerful words that need to be said and heard by everyone. Many people still use the words I love you as a salutation. For example, a person leaving a parent's house after a delicious dinner, might say something like, *"Thanks for dinner, Love Ya,"* as he is walking out the door. If you haven't looked a parent or loved one in the eyes and given them a heartfelt *"I Love You"*, I recommend you start working toward that. For people that have not expressed their feeling much, especially men, it can be quite difficult and even take time to build up to say *"I Love You."*.

Take an opportunity to honor your parents. Schedule a dinner, invite family and close friends and ask each person to say a few words. Hold a family "Roast" on a birthday or anniversary, and share fond memories and humorous occasions. Or, as my wife's family did, on Christmas, make your gift to each other a letter about fond memories. Heck, most people already have enough stuff, and parents can be so hard to shop for anyway. So instead of a present, write a letter of recollection and appreciation, or make a list of your top 10 memories.

In the book Tuesdays with Morrie, Morrie talked about how unfortunate it is that once someone dies, friends start sharing wonderful stories and memories about the person. Morrie questioned why we have to wait to say nice things about a person until they have died. He also indicated how unfortunate it is that the person, about whom the nice things were being said, isn't there to hear them.

Ask Questions

One thing I hear people say all the time, is that they have heard a particular story a hundred times. However, when it comes time to repeat it, they are at a loss for words. If there are stories of significant interest, write them down or videotape your parent delivering her favorite story, so you capture her expressions and mannerisms. Also, as in the case of my parents, do you look at their wedding album without a clue who anyone is? Rather than trying to recall if someone might be a family member, friend, neighbor or business associate, go through photo albums with your parent and write down peoples' names, relationship and places.

If your parent has antiques, collectibles or other items of sentimental value, make sure to ask about the history, significance and even value. Someone once told me that there is a story behind every antique. Do you know the stories associated with your loved one's antiques and collectibles? Remember though, once you ask your parent, make sure to write down what she tells you.

Take the time to document a loved one's life. You'll be amazed at how much you didn't know and how much great stuff you learn. Here's a list of some simple questions to get you started.

- What is something that you always wanted to do, but never have? Why?
- What is something specific that you vividly remember doing as a child?
- Where did you grow up? How did your parent end up there?
- Where did you go to school? What are some fond memories? Do you still keep in touch with any former classmates?
- Who were your best friends at different stages of your life? *(Do you know how to contact them if you need to?)*
- Where are all the places you lived?
- How did you meet mom/dad? Was it love at first site?
- What do you remember most about dating? How long did you date? What kind of things did you do on dates?
- How and when did your dad propose to your mom? Did she say yes right away?
- What is one thing you regret never doing?
- What is most valuable lesson learned in life? What was the situation when you learned it?
- What us your biggest achievement? Why?
- What is your fondest memory? Why?
- What is something that you would like to be remembered for?
- What is something that you would want your great grand children to know about you?

If you are like most people, you will be astonished as to how little you know or are able to recall. Include a resume if possible or other list of work history, military service, honors and recognition, involvement in clubs, organizations, and other affiliations.

This information can also be great to reference when writing an obituary or preparing remarks to celebrate your parent's life at his funeral.

EXERCISE #9 – Memories to Remember	
Places of Residence	
Places of Education	
Military Service & Honors	
Favorite Hobbies	
Club Memberships	
Favorite Song	
Favorite Artist	
Favorite Vacation Spot	
Special Honors or Awards	

Just as many people take photographs on vacations and other events; take your own trip down memory lane with your parent. Reminiscing about the past and fond memories can be great therapy! Think about it. Who do you know that does not like talking about themselves and sharing insight into his life?

Earlier I suggested pulling out a camera and taking pictures or video at an upcoming event. Here is another idea. For your parent's next birthday or anniversary, create a video of his life including sequential pictures from his childhood to the present. Ask a local camera shop about transferring pictures to a video. You can also add his favorite music as background. Not only is this a great present for your parent now, but also a present that you will treasure for life once he has passed on.

Memorialize Life

Create a family tree with your parents. (Trust me, it is a lot easier to do with the input of someone that knows first hand, rather than guessing how pieces fit together.) Even when someone is knowledgeable, it can be difficult to go back more than a generation or two.

If your family has a cemetery plot, you might want to contact the main office at the cemetery to obtain information about each relative that is buried there. Information often includes birth and death dates, cause of death, full name, occupation, and more.

My father always seemed a bit sad on his birthday and I always thought he was having a tough time getting older. Upon his death, we obtained records from the office staff at the cemetery where other family members had been buried. I learned was that my grandfather died two days before my dad's 9th birthday, and was buried on my dad's birthday. While some might be astonished by this story, remember that many older people are very private about their lives, even to their own family. While I knew his dad passed away when he was nine, I did not know the proximity to my dad's birthday or that my grandfather was only in his forties when he passed.

I have provided a worksheet that you might use to begin capturing information. Feel free to create your own worksheet with additional fields for married names, birthdays, city/state where they live(d), cause of death, and location of final resting place. You may quickly find this can be a monumental task if your parent comes from a large family or if "step" relations are involved. Once you have collected the information, the next step may be to create an actual tree diagram. You are on your own for that one.

	MOM's Side	DAD's Side
EXERCISE #10 – Family Tree Information		
Great Grandmother (GGM)		
GGM's Sisters		
GGM's Brothers		
Great Grandfather (GGF)		
GGF's Sisters		
GGF's Brothers		
Grandmother (GM)		
GM's Sisters		
GM's Brothers		
Grandfather (GF)		
GF's Sisters (GFS)		
GFS's children		
GF's Brothers (GFB)		
GFB's children		
Etc.		

Big Picture Considerations

I occasionally hear of siblings that indicate mom or dad wanted me to have this very special (_____you fill in the blank_____). However, two or more siblings are saying the same thing. Whenever possible take steps to avoid sibling conflict. If mom or dad says they want you to have something that carries a significant sentimental value, ask them to state that in a letter to you or suggest it be spelled out in their Will. For any items of sentimental value, I suggest parents indicate their intentions clearly. For example, who should get mom's engagement ring? Dad's coin collection? Bottom line, if there are items that siblings are likely to fight over or feel resentment if they do not get something they feel entitled to, encourage your parents to spell it out in order to avoid conflict. When siblings or relatives live in different parts of the country, this can also help avoid the *"first-come-first-served"* mentality. If a person arrives at a parent's house and starts taking things he or she wants before other family members have a chance to express an interest, it may be too late. Believe it or not this happens.

I was fortunate to receive a few special items from my father, including a watch he received when he graduated from law school, and a painting that he received from a dear friend. Unfortunately, once he passed away and I

240

attempted to share the significance, I found myself unable to recall the specifics around both items. I am now frustrated to realize that I will be unable to share the heritage with my kids. It would have been so easy to write down what he told me.

All too often family members are so physically close to a loved one that they take for granted that they know the intimate details of a loved one's life. Then at such time as you need to write or contribute to the obituary, your mind will invariably be blank. While it is natural to think that you know a tremendous amount about a parent's life, people often do not realize that they were not yet alive during the first twenty or thirty years, and then once born, were too young to recall any details or specifics during until their teenage years. It always seems that the most recent experiences are the memories that are so vivid yet they represent such a small part of a loved one's life.

Summary

As I have repeatedly said throughout this chapter, share your thoughts and feelings while you can, capture memories on film and on paper, and create a legacy that can live on for future generations. Do not take life for granted. Start capturing special memories today and make every interaction count! Be prepared for some good laughs, and tears of joy and sorrow. For that matter, as you recount your parent's life, you may find that you need to resolve an outstanding issue, get an answer to a nagging question, or obtain closure on a matter that has been bothering you for some time. I suggest that you carefully think about any areas of conflict that may cause resentment later if left unresolved. Tremendous healing can occur if you let it. Anything is possible, but you have to make the effort.

KEY LEARNINGS – *Top three learnings from this chapter:*

1.	
2.	
3.	

ACTION ITEMS - *Things you want to do, or do differently:*

Check when Completed	Action Item	Target Completion Date

14

Facing Death

Accepting the fact that your parent has passed away is tough in itself. Combine that with feelings of guilt, sadness, loneliness, agitation and resentment, and you find yourself on an emotional roller coaster. This is normal. This chapter is intended to help you understand what to expect from both death and the grieving process. Depending on your situation, you may want to seek professional counseling.

When a person is faced with the reality of death, family members often start to reprioritize the things they do and the ways they spend their time. For most people dying is a process. Deterioration can be slow or rapid. People are said to handle death in a similar way to how they approach life. Some people want to isolate and approach death in a private manner while others want to be surrounded by loved ones. Some may be more reserved, others more expressive. There is no right way or wrong way. It's up to the person who is dying and it is important to let them die with dignity. Dying involves the physical, emotional and spiritual aspects of a person.

Death is a Reality of Life

Death is one of the toughest realities we all face in life. And dealing with our emotions can be a huge challenge. When faced with the death of a loved one, you have two choices:

1. Mourn the death

2. Celebrate the life

It is my hope that your loved one has lived a long and fulfilling life and you will be able to celebrate the life. While age doesn't make death any easier, it is something people expect as loved ones reach their 70's and 80's.

In the case of a premature or unexpected death, the reality is that you may find yourself mourning the death without choice. Unexpected deaths can be extremely heart-wrenching, as family often hasn't had a chance to prepare or say goodbye. When mourning an abrupt death, it can take time to get over your feelings --whether they are of unfairness, guilt or anger. Regardless of the situation, it takes time to heal wounds.

If your parent has been battling an illness or disease, death can be comforting to know that she has finally been relieved from pain and suffering. Know that no matter what you do, you cannot bring our loved one back to life. As part of the healing process, spend time reflecting on your parent's life, reliving wonderful memories and appreciating the traditions in your family. During these emotional flashbacks, my hope is that more of your tears are of joy instead of sadness.

I lost both of my parents in the last ten years. As I look back, there is something I wish I had done differently. My Dad had been fighting lymphoma leukemia for a couple of years. On his 79th birthday, he became rather delirious after catching what I thought was a common cold. The cold turned out to be pneumonia. Over the next two weeks, he became quite agitated and began doing and saying things that I had never observed before. While I visited him each day, it was very difficult to see him restrained for his own safety. It got to the point where I just couldn't face him in that condition. It was too sad. While I never gave up hope that he would pull through, days later, the doctor called to tell us he would not make it through the night. I chose not to be by his side because I was afraid of death, did not know what to expect and just could not cope. That night he passed away. As I look back, I wish I would have been by his side... holding his hand and telling him how much I loved him.

As for our mother, she had been challenged by dementia for years. She lived in a marvelous facility that specialized in Alzheimer's care and everyone there loved her. On Thanksgiving weekend of 2001, I got the call. She was deteriorating rapidly. When I arrived it was apparent that many of her bodily functions were shutting down. She was on oxygen and was taking huge, gaspy breaths. It was then that I asked my family to leave the room for a minute so that I could have some time alone with her. It was during that three or four minutes that I thanked Mom for a wonderful life. I reflected on a few fond memories, told her that I loved her and I always would, and then I told her that it was okay, almost as if I gave her permission to die. Finally, I told her she was going to a most wonderful place. She immediately began to breathe easier and within minutes, she died at the age of 70. Words cannot describe what a beautiful experience it was to see her released from her suffering. I only wish I had been by my dad's bedside when he died.

I share my story for a couple of reasons:

1. To help you gain perspective to determine what is right for you. If, given the chance to be by your loved one's side, think through what might be right for you.

2. To offer a perspective on death and dying. Prior to my parents' death, I never had any idea of what to expect.

Dealing with Grief

Grief is a natural process people experience over a period of time when they are deprived of a loved one. The death of parent or spouse can be a life-changing experience. It is natural to grieve the death of a loved one before, during and after the actual time of their death. The process of accepting the unacceptable is what grieving is all about.

When a parent or loved one dies, grief will manifest itself in many ways. The following suggests many of the ways people typically grieve. Everyone handles the process differently and that is okay. My pastor indicated that some people often come to him because they do not break down in tears of sadness. Some people become busy managing tasks and details as a way to avoid the reality of death. Others literally may not be able to cope for weeks or months. That is okay, too. Every situation is unique. There is no right way or normal way to feel.

Do not try to rush the grieving process or hold it inside. Get it out. Talk about it with family and friends. When a death occurs, the typical grieving period is six months to a year. Internalizing the pain often makes things worse and prolongs the grieving process. Grief can often be worse or more difficult on dates of significance such as a birthday, wedding anniversary, and the anniversary date of death.

What makes the death of a loved one so hard is that it is not something with which most people have experience. As a result, people do not know what or how to feel. Other things that can complicate death include:

- Not being present when a loved one dies.

- Deaths that occur suddenly, without anticipation or warning.

- Experiencing a traumatic or painful death.

- Deaths that occur after a long illness.

Once you have experienced a death, do not be alarmed by comments that seem insensitive. It will happen. Remember how awkward you were when one of your friends was dealing with a loss and you were not sure what to do or say. I know that when both of my parents died, I felt helpless. I did not know what I should do. My life was turned upside down, yet, the world continued to revolve in spite of my loss.

So why do we grieve? In the book <u>Wild at Heart,</u> John Eldredge states:

> *"It was not your fault and it did matter. Oh what a milestone day that was for me when I simply allowed myself to say that the loss of my father mattered. The tears that flowed were the first I'd ever granted my wound, and they were deeply healing. All those years of sucking it up melted away in my grief. It is so important for us to grieve our wound; it is the only honest thing to do. For in the grieving we admit the truth – that we were hurt by someone we loved, that we lost something very dear, and it hurt us very much. Tears are healing. They help to open and cleanse the wound….. Grief is a form of validation, it says the wound mattered."*

Some people experience grief in many different ways and others only in a few ways. Being at one extreme or the other is OKAY. As you experience the grieving process, I encourage you to seek other resources to help you cope with death. The bookstores are filled with books on the topic of death and dying. To help with your grief, talk with others who have recently lost a loved one. Also talk to your religious leader, family and friends about what you are feeling. As you deem appropriate, you may also choose to talk with a professional counselor.

There are many different types of grief. Some basic forms of grief include:

246

- **Emotional Grief:** Sadness, guilt, loneliness, anger, depression, self-doubt, anxiety, resentment, irritability, etc. Also feelings of hopelessness, helplessness, being overwhelmed, victimized and more.

- **Physical Grief:** Nausea, tears and sobbing, shock, restlessness, exhaustion, inability to sleep, and even wailing.

- **Mental Grief:** Confusion, denial, inability to concentrate, need to rationalize and assess your feelings, sense that you are in a dream and things aren't real, a need for closure, and more.

- **Spiritual Grief:** Renewed or shaken religious beliefs, feeling of being blessed and at peace or feeling of being punished, increased confidence in God or questioning of God, increased prayer and prayer requests, search for answers and explanation, questioning of what happens to someone's soul after death, etc.

- **Social Grief:** A need for isolation or withdrawal, a dependency on family and friends, a rejection or resentment of those offering help and comfort, a need to find distractions, a reluctance to ask others for help, a desire to move somewhere else, etc.

The emotional wounds left by the death take time to heal. It is becoming more and more common for people to participate in "aftercare" activities such as support groups to help them deal with death. You might contact your religious leader or funeral home director to learn about options available in your community.

One word of caution. If you are married or have kids, do not shut them out and carry the entire burden on your shoulders. Children are often more perceptive than we care to admit. They also have a need to understand. There are some great children's books available at local bookstores to help kids when a loved one passes.

What to Do and Who to Call

When a person dies, there are a number of issues that need to be addressed, some that require immediate attention. The following provides insight to the purpose and implications behind many of those tasks. Depending on your religious beliefs, there may be additional considerations not mentioned here. If your loved one has pre-arranged his or her funeral, many of these steps may already be addressed.

1. **Medical Confirmation**: At the time of death, someone of medical background needs to confirm a death has occurred. To do this, a person's vitals will be taken. If your loved one is in a nursing home or medical facility, the staff will confirm the death and work with you to make the necessary arrangements. However, if your loved one dies while at home, regardless of whose home it is, you should call 911. Emergency personnel will come to your house and verify the death and document the person's name, approximate time of death, cause of death, etc. They will also contact the coroner's office and based on the information the authorities provide, the coroner will do one of two things:

    a. If the death appears to be of natural causes and a medical exam is deemed unnecessary, the body will be released to a representative of the funeral home you select. The funeral home will then coordinate the disposition of the body according to the wishes of your family.

    b. If there is any suspicion or uncertainty about the cause of death, the coroner may order the body brought in for an autopsy to determine the cause of death.

2. **Next of Kin Notified**: If you are not present at the time a loved one dies, someone (whether it be a caregiver, nursing home representative, medical facility employee or a public service official) will either call or visit the next of kin to notify them of the death.

3. **Select or Notify Funeral Home:** If you have pre-arranged a funeral or know which funeral home you would like to use, notify the funeral home of the death. If, however, you have not already selected a funeral home, consider these factors:

    - Responsiveness and timely follow-up to your telephone calls. Someone is typically on call 24 hours a day and should be able to return your call promptly.
    - Positive reputation from family members, friends, neighbors, caregivers, place of worship, etc.
    - Licensed
    - Professional designation or affiliation (e.g. National Funeral Directors Association – NFDA or State Association)
    - Availability of professional services, including memorial service assistance, flower arrangements, providing a guest book, submitting the obituary to local newspapers, and more.

4. **Decide on Disposition:** If your loved one's wishes are not known, you may need to decide between earth burial, entombment or cremation. If you are uncertain of your loved one's wishes, you might contact his attorney or your loved one's advance directive documents for clarification. The funeral home will take care of the death certificate and permit for embalmment or cremation. Likewise, they will take care of transporting the body.

5. **Notify Friends and Relatives:** I suggest this step after you contact the funeral home. People usually find that contacting friends and relatives can be an extremely emotional task. Don't hesitate to ask a family friend to make some calls on your behalf.

6. **Notify Your Loved One's Attorney:** This is important for a number of reasons. First, if there is any question of authority, the attorney should have the necessary legal documents (such as a Will) to verify who is appointed as the Executor of the Estate. That person was selected to handle personal matters, including the funeral arrangements. The attorney can also advise of any special wishes, concerns or suggestions. The attorney may also offer to notify you parent's bank, at which point accounts and access to a safety deposit box may be restricted.

7. **Select Location for Memorial Service:** Give consideration to the location of the memorial service. If there is a particular place you'd like to hold the funeral (e.g. church, synagogue, mosque), call to find out the availability of the facility and of a religious leader to perform the ceremony. Coordinate this early so details can be included in the obituary. The important details you will need to provide to the funeral home director include date, time and location of the funeral. This information is also necessary for the obituary.

8. **Designate Organization for Memorials:** People often times designate a cause, such as a non-profit organization, school or foundation, where family and friends can make a memorial contribution in remembrance of your parent. If no organization quickly comes to mind, think about your parent's interest, community involvement, etc. While you might choose to call the organization you select to advise them of their selection, there is no need to do so. They will always be able to locate you via the funeral home to acknowledge and thank you for any gifts. Acknowledgements are typically limited to the name and address of the person making a contribution.

9. **Meet with Funeral Home -** Usually within 24 hours of a death, you will need to meet with the funeral home representative to make arrangements. The funeral director is a valuable resource who serves as advisor and coordinator of the logistical issues. At that time, he will ask for the standard information including full name, address, social security number, place of birth, place of death, military service, and more so he can file the appropriate paper work with county officials. Also, he will require signatures on a number of documents and describe the process over the next few days. Most meetings are approximately one hour in duration. The funeral home is a great resource, so do not hesitate to ask any and all questions you might have. Your funeral director can provide references to community resources and support services to help you as you begin the grieving process.

If you have not pre-planned the funeral, be prepared to discuss the following:

- What is the preferred disposition for the body (*e.g. earth burial, cremation*)
- Would you like to a have a visitation the evening before the actual ceremony?
- Would you like the body to be laid out?
- Who would you like to serve as Pall Bearers?
- Will the family be receiving guests either before or after the service?
- Would you like to a have private service inviting only family and select friends?
- Who from your family will contribute to or write the obituary? How much help do you want/need from the funeral director for this?
- Would you like the funeral home to take care of floral arrangements? If so, do you have any flower preferences?
- Would you like the funeral home to take care of honorariums of the person conducting the memorial service, any musicians or organists, vocalists, etc?
- How many death certificates will you need?
- If an earth burial is planned, does the family already have cemetery plots?

Years ago, I was driving down the road and I saw a bumper sticker that caught my eye. It read "Let's put the FUN back in FUNeral". I couldn't agree more. In fact, my mother passed away a couple of months after I saw the bumper sticker and that is the approach we took. Sure, we went through a grieving process that included crying, being extremely sad, etc. But, to make it a "celebration" of her life, we conjured up and shared the happy and fun memories at her funeral... we even poked a little fun at mom. We know she was laughing up there with us...not slapping our hands. Note: there is a big difference between being disrespectful and having fun. We knew we had successfully celebrated her life in a tactful, upbeat way when those in attendance laughed more than cried. Whichever road you choose is fine. However, just realize that funerals do not have to be somber.

10. **Plan the Memorial Service** – The people that you plan the Memorial Service with will depend on the location you have selected for your Memorial Service. Specifically, if you hold the service at a funeral home, the funeral director may be your best resource. Likewise, if you hold the service at a place of worship, your religious leader will be your best resource. Regardless of the location, consider the following:

- Presence: Will a casket or urn of ashes be present at the service? Would you like to have a large photo of the deceased on the altar or in the front of the room?

- Music/Songs: Are there specific selections you would like played at the service? Also, is there a preference for a vocalist, organ, piano or other musical option?

- Readings: Are there specific readings you'd like...whether from the Bible, favorite poem(s), etc.?

- Perspectives: Whom would you like to speak and offer remarks about the life or character of the deceased? There can be multiple speakers ranging from a worship leader, family member (spouse, son, daughter, aunt, uncle, grandchild, etc.), friend or business associate.

- Location(s): Are you planning a graveside service following a Memorial Service? Will your family be receiving guests before or after the service? Would you like to plan a luncheon or dinner for family, out-of-town guests and other close friends?

If uncertain when planning a service, a great starting point is to request copies of bulletins of other Memorial Services. If not available, create your own mini outline on paper as a good starting point.

If you are reading this section in advance of a loved one's death and think pre-planning arrangements might be appropriate, contact one or more funeral homes to discuss arrangements and make a selection.

Death Certificate

As you might have guessed, a death certificate is similar to a birth certificate. Just as a birth certificate was necessary to obtain a Social Security number, validate identity when enrolling in school, etc., a death certificate is necessary for the following reasons:

- To apply for Social Security Benefits for the surviving spouse
- To apply for retirement funds, deferred salary, accrued vacation pay, unpaid Bonuses, commissions, stock options, etc.
- To initiate a claim and collect on insurance benefits
- To transfer investments (Stocks, Bonds, IRA's, etc.) for estate matters

While four or five death certificates are usually necessary, if a person has not consolidated their financial assets such as stocks and bonds into a managed account, it may be necessary to have individual copies for each institution or company for which assets are held.

When a death occurs, ask your funeral director about any special considerations specific to your city or state. According to an article in the January 17, 2004 edition of the New York Times entitled <u>Death and the City</u>, reporter Wilson H. Beebe Jr. points out that dying in New York City can be challenging. Beebe writes, *"..something must be done with you when you die in New York, and that something requires a document. At some point, your name and Social Security number must cross a Health Department desk. Without a certified death certificate, survivors cannot begin probate on a will, make claims on life insurance policies, apply for Social Security benefits, or perform a host of other tasks involving the business of life."* He continues stating the due to New York's antiquated death registration system, it can take two to six months to get a death certificate. Also, there is only one vital records office in the city. Apparently the City plans to develop an electronic system that will expedite the process, it hasn't set any deadlines.

Facing Death

What to Say

For people who have never experienced death, greeting a family member or friend who has lost a loved one can be quite challenging. Most people simply don't know what to say. Quite often things that are meant to be kind and considerate can be viewed as insensitive or inappropriate. Know that people mean well, even though it may not come across well. While many people make say things like, *"She lived a long life," "He is better off now," "It's going to be okay,"* or *"I know how you must feel,"* can be inappropriate. Instead, comments like *"I'm sorry for your loss," "You are in my prayers,"* or sharing a fond memory can be received much better. Consider asking a question, like *"How are you doing?"* or *"Would you like to get together soon and talk?"* Also, don't refer to the person that died as a he or she. Use the deceased persons name when referring to them.

Families tend to receive a tremendous amount of support (e.g. visits, cards, flowers) over the 7-10 days after death. As a result, the 2-4 weeks after a death is a time when people often struggle the most. It is as this point when friend, neighbors and co-workers are back to life as before. Families find themselves dealing with a number of administrative (e.g. legal and financial) issues at this time. Many people comment that they are still acutely aware of their recent loss, and at the same time are amazed that the world continues to revolve and people are going about day-to-day life.

How to Help

When a death occurs, family members, whether they immediately recognize it or not, may need some assistance. The following is a list of some things that you might consider doing for friend as they experience the death of a loved one. Likewise, these may be things you would like to ask your friends to help with at such time that there is a death in your family.

- Grocery Shopping: Invariably, you will need food, beverages and other supplies. Consider everything from toilet paper and paper products for the kitchen, to snack foods, sandwich items, soft drinks, and coffee.

- Phone Calls: Many people will need to be called and informed when a loved one dies. Decide which people would be appropriate to ask a friend to contact on your behalf to notify them of the death and funeral arrangements.

- Preparing for Guests: If you expect people to be coming in from out of town, give consideration to transportation and lodging arrangements. Also, as people may be dropping by your house, maybe you would like to ask a friend to help you clean your house so it is presentable for company.

Acknowledge Gifts and Flowers

Much like you appreciate receiving a thank-you note from a friend or family member following a kind gesture on your part, you will want to be sure to send a note to all those who sent flowers, made a donation, prepared food or put forth any other kind gesture or gift.

Big Picture Considerations

At a time when a person is dying, the family is often called upon to discuss his wishes and confirm any advance directives. This includes issues such as resuscitation orders, surgery options and desire to transport to a hospital or make him as comfortable as possible in his current environment. Just know that there are no right or wrong answers. Also, look to any medical staff that is available for advice and considerations.

An often overlooked, yet challenging aspect of death is handling the disposition of a loved one's personal items. One man's junk is another man's treasures. It can be quite difficult to dispose of a loved one's possessions. Families often invite friends over to pick and choose items before items are offered for sale or consignment. Most of us have accumulated a lot of stuff over the years. Maybe it's time to start eliminating stuff slowly over time. Practically speaking, you're leaving a lot of work to the surviving family members. Spiritually speaking, you can't take it with you and people will not remember you for your possessions. According to a local dealer who has handled thousands of estates over the years, there are stages that family members go through. Initially, there is a disposal of stuff but keeping special items that were near and dear to your loved one (e.g. a special antique, piece of art work, a vase, photos, etc.) Then after about three years, there is another disposal of things you're now able to let go of things that have sat in your basement unused for a period of time.

If you've lost a loved one (e.g. parent, spouse, aunt/uncle, sibling), it can be extremely difficult to feel optimistic about the future. And unless your friends or family has been through a similar situation, chances are they are not going to understand the deep hurt you feel. Also, when the funeral or memorial service is over and you think you can finally relax, you realize that there is a lot more to do. There are estate matters that will need to be addressed, arrangement will need to be made for a grave stone, thanks are typically sent to people for their flowers and gifts and don't forget about the tax return that will need to be filed for any income earning or received during your parent's final year.

Summary

End-of-life should not be a lonely, painful or traumatic experience for people and their families. Always strive to ensure a person is comfortable and maintains his dignity.

Everyone responds to aging, illness and death differently. For an older person, factors that often play a significant role include their previous exposure to death, their faith or religious belief system, and their personality. Common reactions often include:

- Acceptance or denial
- Peace or anger
- Calm, fear or even guilt

While your parent is living, regardless of his medical condition, treat him with the same dignity and respect as you always have. As such, his opinion still counts, so keep asking for it. He still has feelings, so do not exclude him. He has years and years of wisdom, so share life stories with him and seek his counsel and advice. Your thoughtfulness and tact will help him realize that you even coming to him to discuss issues is a sign you love him.

Know that everyone grieves differently. Many people need time and space before there are able to jump back into everyday life. Remember that there is not right or wrong way. Also, don't be afraid to seek professional counseling. When our Mother died, I came to realize that I was all-alone and for the first time in my life totally responsible for everything I did. While our Mother did not recognize us during her last year or two due to her dementia, for some reason it was different once she passed away. I found myself depressed and realized that I has issues or concerns that I had never acknowledged but needed to be addressed. Also, in addition to taking care of yourself, don't neglect your family. Often people fail to recognize that other family members are also impacted directly and indirectly from a death.

KEY LEARNINGS – *Top three learnings from this chapter:*

1.

2.

3.

ACTION ITEMS - *Things you want to do, or do differently:*

Check when Completed	Action Item	Target Completion Date

#15

Closing Comments

I sincerely hope that the material presented throughout this Resource Guide prepares you for the journey ahead and that you are now better able to make informed decisions. I encourage you to act and apply your new knowledge to make a difference in someone's life.

Please recommend **<u>The Caregiver Resource Guide</u>** to your family, friends, neighbors and co-workers. As I mentioned in the opening chapter, everyone will be impacting by caregiving at some point in their life. Copies of this Resource Guide are available for purchase on my website – www.AgingUSA.com and at many bookstores across the country.

If I can be of assistance, my contact information is available on my website - www.AgingUSA.com. I pray that your journey will be rewarding. Let me close by sharing excerpts from an e-mail that I received in 2002 that I understand may have originally been written by Andy Rooney.

I'VE LEARNED....
- That being kind is more important than being right.
- That I can always pray for someone when I don't have the strength to help him in some other way.
- That sometimes all a person needs is a hand to hold and a heart to understand.
- That under everyone's hard shell is someone who wants to be appreciated and loved.
- That the Lord didn't do it all in one day. What makes me think I can?
- That to ignore the facts does not change the facts.
- That I can't choose how I feel, but I can choose what I do about it.

#16

Key Terms and Definitions

In this section, I provide explanations of common terms that are often associated with aging. Chances are you will frequently see many of these terms.

TERM	DEFINITION / EXPLANATION
AARP	The AARP is a nonprofit, nonpartisan membership organization for people 50 and over. AARP provides information and resources; advocate on legislative, consumer, and legal issues; assist members to serve their communities; and offer a wide range of unique benefits, special products, and services for members. AARP offers a number of Member Benefits provided by third parties through contractual arrangements with a subsidiary of AARP. AARP Membership Benefits currently available to AARP Members include: life, auto and homeowner's insurance; discounts on products and services, on-line resources, and publications.
Adult Day Care	Enrichment programs typically offered at a Senior or Community Center that provide senior citizens with social, educational and recreational programs. Transportation and meals are often provided.
Advance Directives	Legal documents executed by a mentally competent person that indicates his medical wishes should it be necessary for someone else to make treatment decisions on his behalf.

Age in Place	Refers to people growing old in the home where they currently live.
Agent	Someone appointed by your parent, usually a trusted family member or friend that is authorized by a Power of Attorney to make legal decisions on his or her behalf.
Agitation	Disruptive behavior such as screaming, shouting, cursing, moaning, and fidgeting that interferes in the well being of others
Alzheimer's Disease	A progressive disease characterized by intellectual challenges that are a disruption of functioning such as thinking, remembering and reasoning.
Annual Exclusions	Each calendar year, a person can transfer or gift tax-free amounts of up to and including $11,000 to others.
Arthritis	A disease commonly associated with pain and stiffness in joints
Assessment	An evaluation of a person's medical, mental, emotional, and social capabilities.
Assisted Living Facility	A residential care setting that provides housing, meals, activities, and various support services for seniors needing a little extra assistance for things like dispensing medication and assistance with personal care such as bathing, grooming and dressing.
Autonomy	A person's ability to act in her own best interest
Autopsy	Medical examination of a body after death, usually to determine the cause of death.
Behavioral Symptoms	Physical and emotional symptoms such as wandering, depression, anxiety and hostility.

Beneficiary	An individual named in a will who is designated to receive all or part of an estate upon someone's death.
Bereavement	The process of dealing with or grieving over a death.
Cancer	A group of many related diseases all of which involve out-of-control growth and spread of abnormal cells in any of the body's tissues.
Caregiver	Persons with primary responsibility for the care and well being of an elderly or incapacitated person. Caregivers are typically a family member or a designated health care provider.
Case Management	A term used by care professionals that indicates a person's medical condition, care requirements and actions to meet his needs.
Coexisting Illness	Multiple medical conditions that simultaneously exist with one another, such as diabetes and high blood pressure.
Cognitive Abilities	Mental abilities such as judgment, memory, learning, comprehension, and reasoning.
Competency	A person's ability to make informed choices.
Continuum of Care	Refers to the ability to provide uninterrupted levels of care throughout the progression of a person's illness, providing more or less care as appropriate.
Coordination of Benefits	The process of ensuring medical claims are paid appropriately when a person has multiple providers of health care coverage.
Co-payment	Typically a flat dollar amount that the recipient must pay based on the medical services received.
Covered Expenses	The medical procedures or services that a member's health care plan will pay.

Cueing	Providing someone direction such as instruction or hints to assist a person who is experiencing memory difficulties.
Curative Care	Care intended to treat or cure a person's illness with the intent to maximizing someone's life.
Custodial Care	Basic care such as bathing, dressing, and grooming that can be given safely and reasonably by a person who is not medically skilled.
DNR	Do Not Resuscitate – an order not to perform life saving measures when a person's heart stops or he stops breathing.
Death Certificate	A document signed by a doctor that confirms a person's death and is required to handle estate matters.
Deductible	An amount payable by person before her insurance begins to pay for medical services.
Deficits	Physical and/or cognitive abilities that have deteriorated or a person has lost as a result of aging or a medical condition.
Dementia	The loss or deterioration of intellectual functions (such as thinking, remembering, and reasoning) that interfere with a person's daily living. Dementia is not a disease itself. Rather it is a group of symptoms. Symptoms may include changes in personality, mood, and behavior. Dementia is irreversible when caused by disease or injury.
Detachment	The recognition that we are not responsible for another person's medical condition, treatment and decisions. Also, the emotional separation from another person so that we are not used, abused or manipulated by others actions or inactions.
Diagnosis	The process whereby a physician determines a person's medical condition by studying the patient's

	medical history, symptoms, examining the patient, and analyzing the results of any tests performed.
Dignity	Avoiding degrading actions or words to preserve a person's self-respect.
Durable Power of Attorney	A legal document that authorizes an agent (usually a trusted family member or friend) to make legal decisions on the person's behalf when unavailable or unable to do so himself.
Durable Power of Attorney for Health Care	A legal document that appoints an agent to make decisions regarding health care, including choice of health care providers, medical treatment, and end-of-life decisions.
Elder Law Attorney	An attorney who practices or specializes in the legal issues primarily pertaining to older adults.
Executor	The individual named in a will who manages the estate of a deceased individual according to their wishes.
Estate Planning	A process of assessing a person's accumulated wealth and making decisions to preserve assets and to minimize taxes in the eventual transfer of their assets to others.
Estate Tax	A federal tax on a person's assets at the time of death above a certain dollar amount.
Exclusions	Medical services or procedures that are not covered by a person's medical insurance plan.
Functional Assessment	An evaluation to identifying areas where a person is functioning below the norm and to identify challenges that may impede a person's ability to independently care for herself and function in everyday society.

Funeral Pre-Planning	A process of making your wishes and intentions known regarding your funeral prior to your death.
Gait	Refers to how a person walks, including their speed, balance and ability to lift her feet as she walks.
Geriatric Functional Assessment	SEE Functional Assessment.
Geriatrics	A general term referring to issues involving older people.
Geriatrician	A medical doctor specializing in the care of older adults.
Grief	An emotion exhibited by people who have suffered a great loss often characterized by sobbing, wailing, and the temporary ability to clearly reason.
Hallucination	A sensory experience whereby a person sees, hears, smells, tastes, or feels something that isn't there.
Heart Disease	A general medical term referring to cardiovascular dysfunction usually associated with a heart attack.
Hoarding	An obsessive behavior whereby a person collects (stockpiles) things often of little or no value and then hides or guards them.
HMO	Health Maintenance Organization offering medical insurance.
Home Health Care	A range of nursing and homemaker services provided to persons in their home as needed.
Honorarium	A payment for a service for which a price is not set.
Hospice	A philosophy and approach to providing comfort and care to people with a terminal disease and short life expectancy.

Huntington Disease	A degenerative brain disorder that slowly reduces an individual's ability to walk, think, talk and reason.
Incontinence	Loss of control over bladder or bowel function.
Independent Living	Refers to a living environment, similar to an apartment, for more active seniors where services such as meals, activities, transportation, housekeeping and security are available.
In-Home Care	See HOME HEALTH CARE.
Legacy	Maintaining an historical record of a person and events of her life for future generations to enjoy.
Living Trust	A legal document governed by a trustee (usually a trusted friend, family member, or bank representative) that proves stipulations on how one's assets are to be managed while in trust and distributed upon death.
Living Will	A legal document expressing a person's decision on the use of artificial life support systems.
Long Term Care	Care provided on an ongoing basis to provide for a person's needs including adult day care, in-home care, nursing home care, and hospice care.
Long Term Care Insurance	Insurance that pays for a person's care arrangements after certain criteria and eligibility requirements are met. Often the coverage period or maximum payout is defined.
Managed Care	Care services covered by an HMO medical insurance plan.
Meals on Wheels	A community service that delivers meals to homebound elderly people.

Medicaid	A federal government program administered by states that provides health care and related services to low-income individuals.
Medicare	A federal health insurance program for people age 65 and older.
Medicare Eligible Expenses	Expenses for medical procedures and services recognized and approved by Medicare and provided by doctors that accept Medicare for payment.
Needs	Issues of critical importance to one's health, well-being and safety.
NORC	An acronym standing for Naturally Occurring Retirement Community. A neighborhood not originally planned for senior citizens but where most of its residents have grown old.
Nursing Care	A residential care setting that provides housing, meals, activities, and various support services for seniors including medical assistance by trained nurses aides, LPN's and RN's.
Obituary	A brief article that appears in newspapers and acknowledges a person's death, indicates arrangements and briefly recaps significant events, contributions or achievements of a person's life.
Osteoporosis	A medical condition where the amount of calcium in a person's bones decreases resulting in frequent fractures and a stooped posture.
Palliative Care	Care designed to make a patient comfortable when suffering from a terminal, illness.
Paranoia	Unprovoked or unexplainable suspicion of others.

Parkinson's Disease	A disorder of the central nervous system, commonly seen as uncontrollable tremor or shaking.
Personal Care	Refers to issues such as grooming, bathing, continence, dressing, taking medication nutrition, management of money and the like.
Pillaging	An obsessive behavior whereby a person takes things, often of little or no value, that belong to someone else, often thinking it is hers.
Power of Attorney	See DURABLE POWER OF ATTORNEY.
Pre-Need	See FUNERAL PRE PLANNING.
Probate	The disclosure and settlement of deceased person's estate whereby the county government accounts for and validates the legitimacy of any advance directive or handles the distribution of one's assets according to state law.
Quality Care	Term used to describe a level of care and services provided to a person in a dignified, gentle and caring manner.
Reassurance	Encouragement often provided to a person as a means to relieve fear, anxiety, tension, and confusion that can result from deteriorating cognitive abilities.
Reinforcement	The use of praise, encouragement and repetition to help preserve a person's memory, capabilities, and level of self-confidence.
Repetitive Behaviors	The constant repeating of questions, concerns or physical behaviors, common in people with dementia.
Respite	A rejuvenating break or time away from the constant demands on a person providing caregiver services.

Respite Care	Temporary caregiver services that provide a primary caregiver with short-term relief (e.g., in-home assistance, short nursing home stays, adult day care).
Restraints	Devices used to restrict and control a person's movement for the purpose of ensuring the safety of the person and those around them.
Retirement Living	Independent living provided in a community dedicated to providing carefree and secure living for senior citizens.
Rigidity	Tightness or increase in muscle tone at rest – stiffness.
Senior Centers	Facilities offering supervised recreational, educational and social programs for people ages 55 and older.
Senior Managed Care	Health care services offered by an insurance company or HMO specific to the needs of senior citizens.
Sequencing	Refers to doing things or completing tasks in a logical, predictable order.
Shadowing	Behavior commonly associated with following, mimicking, and interrupting people.
Skilled Nursing Care	A residential care setting providing a level of care that includes ongoing more advanced medical or nursing services including the needs of someone confined to a bed or wheelchair.
Social HMO	An emerging Age in Place alternative currently in the pilot or test stage providing various social services, housekeeping, medical, visiting nurses, transportation, home delivered meals and skilled services that enable a person to remain living at home.

Social Security	Services provided by the federal government that include retirement benefits, survivor benefits, Medicare, Disability and Family benefits to elderly or disabled people.
Social Worker	Someone trained and dedicated to the care and well being of an elderly person or other clientele.
Special Care Unit	Designated areas or units within a residential care facility or nursing home providing care to address a specific need such as Dementia or other advanced medical conditions.
Stages	Progression of a disease defined by levels or periods of severity: early, mild, moderate, or severe.
Sundowning	An unsettled behavior or agitation that commonly occurs in the late afternoon or early evening.
Support Group	Facilitated gathering of family, friends, or others with a common interest, often a loved one suffering from a common illness, for the purpose of discussing issues related to the illness, and sharing hope, strength and experience.
Supplemental Health Insurance	Insurance that pays towards approved services that are not covered or only partially covered by a primary insurance.
Trust	A legal entity established to hold ownership of property and assets on behalf of a personal or family estate.
Trustee	The individual or bank managing the assets of the living trust.
Unified Credit	Refers to a lump sum amount that can be transferred to another person tax-free. The unified credit amount for 2004 and 2005 is $1,500,000.

Validation	Giving approval to other's thoughts and emotion by sharing questions, concerns and experiences with them to help them through difficult times.
Wandering	A behavior commonly associated with dementia whereby people stray from a familiar surrounding and often become lost.
Wants	Things that people have become accustomed to and tend to desire but that are not critical to one's health, well-being and safety.
Will	A legal document that names a person to manage the estate according to the document and addresses the desired disposition of someone's accumulated wealth and personal items.

For information on
Aging America Resources
or to order additional copies of
The Caregiver Resource Guide,
visit us in the web at
www.AgingUSA.com
or **www.CareMinistry.com.**